HOW TO SAVE BIG BUCK$
ON YOUR PET'S VETERINARY BILLS

Additional titles by Alan W. Mac Carthy, Jr., D.V.M.

Available from First-Care! Company

An Owner's Guide to Emergency Care for Dogs

An Owner's Guide to Emergency Care for Cats

First-Care! Company
Post Office Box 427
Pala, California 92059

HOW TO SAVE BIG BUCK$ ON YOUR PET'S VETERINARY BILLS

*****

ALAN W. MAC CARTHY, JR., D.V.M.

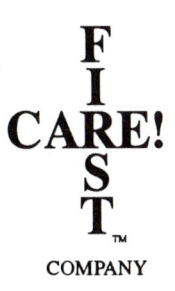

FIRST CARE! COMPANY

A FIRST-CARE! COMPANY PUBLICATION

1992

A First-Care! Book
Published by First-Care! Company Publications
Copyright © 1992 by Alan W. Mac Carthy, Jr. CORP.
All rights reserved.

No part of this book may be reproduced or utilized in any form or by any means, electronic or mechanical including photostat, xerography, microfilm, or by any information storage and retrieval system without the express written permission of Alan W. Mac Carthy, Jr. CORP., Post Office Box 427, Pala, California 92059 U.S.A.

Disclaimer

Alan W. Mac Carthy, Jr. CORP., First-Care! Company, First-Care! Company Publications, and Alan W. Mac Carthy, Jr., D.V.M. assume no responsibility for any injury or damages resulting from the use of any information included in this book.

ISBN 1-882822-00-5
Printed in the United States of America

First Printing: December 1992

TABLE OF CONTENTS

INTRODUCTION 1
CHAPTER 1: A Trip To The Veterinarian 5
    Your Veterinarian 5
    The Veterinary Facility 6
    The Appointment 6
    The Office Call 8
    The Examination 9
    The Consultation 10
        The Diagnosis 10
        The Treatment Plan 12
        The Estimate 13
    The Bill 15
    Cost Worksheet 17
CHAPTER 2: Understanding The Estimate 18
    Hospitalization Charges 18
    Laboratory and X-ray Charges 21
    Dispensed Medication Charges 26
CHAPTER 3: Finances 30
    Expense Limits 30
    Alternate Treatment Plans 32
    Financial Arrangements 35
    Financial Problems 38
CHAPTER 4: Second Opinions 40
CHAPTER 5: Don't Let Little Problems Grow 45
CHAPTER 6: Avoid After Hours Emergencies 48
    Twenty-four Hour Veterinary Facilities 48
    Emergency Pet Clinics 49
    Regular Veterinary Facilities 50
CHAPTER 7: Vaccinations 56
    Regular Veterinary Office 56
    Vaccination Clinics 60
    Do-It-Yourself Kits 61

CHAPTER 8: Spaying and Neutering 63
    Comparison Shopping..... 65
    Spay and Neuter Clinics 66
    Non-Profit Organizations. 67
    Third Party Assistance 68
    Post-Surgical Complications........ 68
CHAPTER 9: Money Saving Health Tips.. 69
    Tips for Both Dogs and Cats........ 69
    Tips Specifically for Dogs 72
    Tips Specifically for Cats. 75
CHAPTER 10: Things To Do At Home..... 77
    Books and Manuals........ 77
    Telephone Advice.......... 78
        Your Own Veterinarian's Staff...... 79
        Emergency Facility Staff 81
        Breeders 83
    Preventive Measures....... 83
    Basic Emergency Kit 86
CHAPTER 11: Other Businesses 87
    Groomers......... 87
    Boarding Kennels 88
    Pet Sitters......... 88
    Exterminators.... 88
CHAPTER 12: Other Suppliers.... 90
    Pet Supplies...... 90
    Dog Foods 91
    Cat Foods......... 92
    Special Diets 93
CHAPTER 13: Miscellaneous Tips 94
CHAPTER 14: Client Dissatisfaction........ 96

APPENDIX A: Poison Control Centers..... 103
APPENDIX B: Boards of Veterinary Medicine........ 107
APPENDIX C: Colleges and Universities 111

INTRODUCTION

I wish I could assure you that your pet, dog or cat, will live a long, comfortable, and healthy life. However, after practicing small animal medicine for over twenty-five years, I have learned that, no matter how much we wish otherwise, real life all too often includes injury and disease. The cars on the road are real, the poisons in your home are real, and the viruses floating around in the air your pet breathes are real. Injuries and diseases are going to happen no matter how protective you are, and when they do, you are going to need the services of a veterinarian. My purpose in writing this book is to describe for you proven ways of avoiding veterinary medical problems, and to reveal to you some sensible ways to get through those that are inevitable as economically as possible.

When I retired from my small animal practice, I founded the **FIRST-CARE! COMPANY** to manufacture and sell veterinary first-aid and emergency kits for cat and dog owners, and to publish the books and manuals which would allow me to share the medical knowledge I had gained over the years. I wrote this book, *How to Save BIG BUCK$ on Your Pet's Veterinary Bills,* as a companion to the books, *An Owner's Guide to Emergency Care for Dogs* and *An Owner's Guide to Emergency Care for Cats*. While I was writing the emergency care books, I frequently thought about how expensive veterinary medicine can be when a pet is severely hurt or becomes seriously ill. Consequently, I decided to write a book exploring various methods of saving money on veterinary costs. While this started out to concern only emergencies, it soon became apparent the principles could be expanded to cover all aspects of veterinary medicine.

I had three goals in mind when I wrote this book. The first was to emphasize the importance of preventing injury and illness, and to show how such prevention can be most economically obtained. Secondly, I wanted to emphasize the importance of knowledge in saving money. Knowledge allows you to avoid expensive professional help when it is not needed. Finally, I wanted to emphasize the fact that veterinary medicine is a business and, as business people as well as doctors, veterinarians are generally open to negotiations concerning treatment plans and finances. These negotiations have made it financially possible for some pet owners to have their pet treated instead of being "put to sleep"—permanently.

The proper application of prevention can save you **BIG BUCK$**. If the only times you go to your veterinarian are for preventive services such as vaccinations, neutering surgery, and physical exams, it is difficult to overspend your veterinary medicine budget. A very important money saving tip is to spend money and see your veterinarian for the preventive medical services he or she offers. Preventive medicine is, and always will be, the least expensive medicine available. Prevention, however, involves more than just preventive medicine. There are other preventive steps, described in this book, which require certain actions on your part to help safeguard your pet's health.

Basic health care knowledge is another important money saving aid. Each pet owner should know what constitutes sickness and what constitutes health. This knowledge is necessary when considering how to save **BIG BUCK$**, because you don't want to be in your veterinarian's office if you don't need to be. For example, there is no reason to rush to your veterinarian because your four months old dog or cat just lost a tooth—all puppies and kittens loose their "baby" teeth at approximately this age—or if your pet vomits once or twice after eating too much too fast. Buy medical information books about your pet's health, or save money by checking such books out of your local library and making appropriate notes. Pet health books can save you hundreds of dollars in veterinary medical expenses. Once you have decided something is abnormal, the next step is to decide whether it needs to be treated as an emergency. This subject is discussed in detail in my books, ***An Owner's Guide to Emergency Care for Cats*** and ***An Owner's Guide to Emergency Care for Dogs***. If you want to save money on your veterinary costs, you need this knowledge.

Together with prevention and knowledge, you must occasionally use negotiation as a means of reducing your veterinary costs. Your goal is to find a combination of a diagnostic plan, treatment plan, and payment plan you can afford. As long as you realize that curtailing diagnostic procedures will reduce the accuracy of your veterinarian's diagnosis which, in turn, may reduce the efficacy of your veterinarian's treatment plan, you and your veterinarian can find a compromise treatment plan in almost every illness or injury.

What is a large veterinary bill for a dog or cat? While costs vary according to geography, a large bill for a single sickness or injury would be between one and two thousand dollars, especially if an emergency clinic was involved. Occasionally, the cost of treating a prolonged illness or repairing severe structural damage could be three thousand dollars, or even more. I mention these figures only for your consideration. If spending this amount of money on your pet's health needs is within your budget, would cause no financial hardship to you or your family, and can be accepted as the price you must sometimes pay for the privilege of owning a dog or cat, you probably don't need the information contained in this book. I wrote this book for pet owners who have some financial limitations on the amount they can spend on veterinary fees, but who are, within limits, able and willing to stretch the family budget on occasion to both fix and keep their pets healthy.

ALAN W. MAC CARTHY, JR., D.V.M.

CHAPTER 1:

A TRIP TO THE VETERINARIAN

Before getting into specific money saving ideas, I want to briefly introduce you to your veterinarian, his or her facility, and what you should expect when you need your veterinarian's services.

YOUR VETERINARIAN

Your veterinarian, like your physician, spends an average of four years in college before being admitted to veterinary medical school, which takes four additional years. After graduation from veterinary medical school, a veterinarian has to take a series of comprehensive examinations to prove to an examining board in their State that they are competent to practice veterinary medicine before the examining board will issue them a license. Each veterinarian's license should be available for your inspection wherever a veterinarian works. Some States issue temporary licenses, but these also must be available for inspection. In every State, it is against the law to practice veterinary medicine or dentistry without a license. State veterinary examining boards also have the power to suspend or revoke a veterinarian's license if they determine a veterinarian is no longer practicing in a safe, legal, and knowledgeable manner.

$ *TIP: While State laws prevent the practice of veterinary medicine without a license, they do not prevent you from medically treating your own dog or cat, as long as you do it in a humane fashion.*

THE VETERINARY FACILITY

A typical veterinary facility has many parts. These include: a waiting room, a receptionist or business area, and one or more examination rooms. These are the areas called the public areas. The medical (non-public) areas consist of treatment facilities, surgical and recovery areas, kennel areas, laboratory facilities, and x-ray facilities. Larger or specialized practices may have additional medical areas to meet specific needs.

A veterinarian can give a veterinary facility any name he or she desires. There is no implied meaning to the names "medical center," "hospital," or "clinic." They are simply the names someone has chosen, and are used interchangeably. The names do not imply level of care, open hours, size of facility, or fees charged. A "clinic" may charge very high fees, and a "medical center" may be comparatively inexpensive. A "hospital" can exist in a small shopping center store, and a "clinic" may occupy a multiple story building.

THE APPOINTMENT

Always telephone your veterinarian's facility in advance to make an appointment. Even in the case of an emergency, a telephone call to make an appointment is very important. Do not just get into the car, go, and expect to find a veterinarian available. There are occasions when your veterinarian is not available, even when the hospital or clinic is open. There are times when emergency facilities are not open, or a veterinarian is not present, or when they are so busy they cannot take another emergency. By calling first, you will give your veterinarian or emergency facility the opportunity to refer you to another location on those rare occasions when they cannot be of assistance.

Information should be shared while making an appointment. You should give the receptionist a summary of your pet's symptoms, including body temperature. This will allow the receptionist to schedule an appointment that is appropriate for your pet's condition. Early morning appointments can frequently save money. If sedation or general anesthesia is required, an early morning appointment may allow sufficient recovery time to avoid the expense of overnight hospitalization. If laboratory blood work might be required, an appointment can be scheduled before the daily pickup time if your veterinarian uses an outside laboratory. Your description of your pet's medical problem may suggest that time is important, and, if so, the receptionist will tell you to come in immediately. True emergencies can almost always be squeezed into a busy schedule. You might have to wait a while before the doctor can personally talk with you, but your pet will be seen almost as soon as you arrive. During your phone call to make an appointment, the receptionist can tell you if there is anything you should bring to the appointment, such as a fecal sample or urine sample. If you are new to the practice, this is also the time you should ask for information concerning fees and financial policies. If you anticipate using a credit card, make sure your veterinarian accepts them. If you are planning to be billed for the visit, make sure your veterinarian offers credit. Many only offer credit to clients who have made prior arrangements and filled out a credit application form. Since billing is both time consuming and expensive most veterinarians request payment when the services are rendered.

When you arrive at your veterinarian's facility make sure your dog or cat is completely under control. For dogs, this means a leash, harness, or sturdy carrier. For cats, a sturdy carrier is best. There have been many instances when an unleashed or uncrated pet got loose in a veterinary facility parking lot, ran into the street, and either got injured by a passing car or disappeared into unknown parts of a strange neighborhood. Unleashed dogs may also run up to another dog just arriving or leaving the facility and may either get bitten or exposed to some contagious disease. Unrestrained cats can become so terrified during the car ride that they decide to hide under the car seats. I have had concerned cat owners literally take their cars apart, in my hospital parking lot, trying to find their cat who has hidden inside the car seat springs.

THE OFFICE CALL

Shortly after arriving, clients and patients are escorted to an examination room. In most veterinary facilities you will be called the client and your pet will be called the patient. If you have made an appointment and arrived on time, the shortly mentioned above should be very short. I like to see signs in waiting rooms that say if you have been waiting for more than ten minutes to please let someone know. I especially like the ones that say that if you have been kept waiting for more than fifteen minutes you will receive a discount, but you don't see many of these. In many families today both adult members work, so going to a veterinarian frequently means someone has to take time off from work. While the visit to the veterinarian may be unavoidable, to be kept waiting is going to cost you **BIG BUCK$** in lost income and is unexcusable. Yes, emergencies happen and if, when you arrive, the receptionist explains that an emergency has arisen and the doctor is going to be late with the appointment schedule, you have no real choice but to accept the situation. You can choose to wait, or you can reschedule the appointment. These situations can usually be avoided by calling your veterinarian's office shortly before your appointment time to find out if the doctor is seeing appointments on schedule. Emergency facilities are different because they deal exclusively with emergencies. If, when you arrive at an emergency facility, you are told that the wait is two hours, don't assume that you will be seen in two hours, since emergencies are seen in order of severity instead of first come, first seen. *If, while waiting at an emergency clinic, you notice all the other patients, even recent arrivals, are being seen before you, you might want to reexamine your reason for being there.*

THE EXAMINATION

When the doctor comes into the examination room, things start to happen. From a financial point of view, you are now going to be charged for an office call and examination. Even if you decide you want no further treatment, you will still be charged an office call and examination fee. *This is an expensive way to discover that there is nothing wrong with your pet, and you shouldn't be there at all.* While physically examining your dog or cat, the veterinarian will ask questions concerning the injury or illness. This is called taking a history. Don't bend the facts because of embarrassment or fear of reprisal. If your pet has been sick for a week, don't tell the veterinarian that he or she just got sick last night. You may feel badly for waiting so long to seek help, but don't hinder your veterinarian's ability to make a diagnosis by giving false information. If your pet is not current on his or her vaccinations, say so. You need to help your veterinarian in every way possible. When the clinical symptoms do not agree with the facts you provide, your veterinarian may hesitate before making a final diagnosis, and this may mean more tests, and additional expense to you. If, for example, you indicate that your dog's distemper vaccinations are up to date and this is not true, even if your dog has distemper, your veterinarian may rule it out as a diagnosis until all other possibilities have been exhausted.

THE CONSULTATION

This is when your veterinarian talks to you about your pet's case. Once your veterinarian has completed the examination, he or she is going to give you a lot of information in a short time. How you handle this information is extremely important. In just a few minutes, you are going to be given either a diagnosis or a diagnostic plan (an outline of what needs to be done to arrive at a diagnosis), a treatment plan, and an estimate of costs.

The Diagnosis

Once your veterinarian has taken a history and discovered the clinical symptoms, there are two types of diagnoses that he or she can make:

1. **Presumptive Diagnosis:** This is your veterinarian's number one suspicion, and is made whenever your veterinarian is unable, without further testing, to make a final diagnosis. The following are examples of presumptive diagnoses and the tests that might be recommended as part of the diagnostic plan:

PRESUMPTIVE DIAGNOSIS	TEST
Broken Leg	X-rays
Anemia	Red Blood Count
Bacterial Infection	White Blood Count
Skin Cancer	Surgical Biopsy
Kidney Failure	Blood Chemistry
Ear Infection	Bacterial Culture
Feline Leukemia	Antibody Testing

    The list, of course, goes on and on, but the important thing is to carefully consider the consequences. If the cost of the diagnostic plan approaches or exceeds your established expense limits (see page 30), you may not be able to afford a primary or alternate treatment plan once the final diagnosis is made. If your veterinarian is unable to make an immediate final diagnosis, you need to know what the final diagnosis possibilities are, and how much the diagnostic plan needed to make a final diagnosis is going to cost. Additionally, you will need to know how much the treatment for each of the final diagnosis possibilities is likely to cost. The reason you need this information immediately is that there may be valid financial reasons for not spending two hundred dollars on diagnostic x-rays and laboratory work if you cannot afford to spend the additional six hundred dollars on treatment, if your veterinarian's suspicion is confirmed. For example, your veterinarian may suspect your pet has a broken leg and advises that a sedative be given and x-rays taken at a cost of $80.00. If you can only afford a total of $150.00, the $50.00 left over, after paying $20.00 for the office call/examination and $80.00 for the sedative and x-rays, will not pay for very much repair work.

$ TIP: *If you would be financially unable to afford the treatment if the presumptive diagnosis turns out to be accurate, you are probably financially unable to afford the tests, x-rays, or surgery necessary to make a final diagnosis.*

2. **Final Diagnosis:** When a certain set of symptoms can mean more than one thing, it is very natural, and medically proper, for your veterinarian to want to rule out all but one of the possible problems, arriving at a final diagnosis. Only after arriving at a final diagnosis will your veterinarian be able to recommend a primary treatment plan, alternate treatment plans, a minimal treatment plan, and tell you what the prognosis (outcome) is likely to be.

At the end of this chapter, on page 17, I have included a worksheet outlining the questions you might want to ask your veterinarian during this time. Only by knowing what needs to be done, and the costs involved, to go from a presumptive diagnosis to a final diagnosis, and by knowing the costs involved in the treatment of the suspected final diagnosis, including aftercare, can you make the necessary financial decisions. This worksheet takes you, step by step, through each of the above stages to give you the estimated final cost of your pet's problem, which is an amount you can compare with any expense limitations you have set.

The Treatment Plan

Once your veterinarian has made a final diagnosis, he or she will suggest a treatment plan. You should assume that this plan is for the best—and probably most expensive—approach to the problem. This is proper, but at this point many pet owners make critical decisions based on insufficient information. If you are given an estimate of seven hundred fifty dollars for applying a bone plate to your pet's broken leg, and that amount is well above your financial limits, don't automatically consider euthanasia as the only other option. Ask for less expensive alternate treatment plans (see page 32). The cost of these alternate treatment plans should also be entered into the worksheet. By comparing the cost of the primary treatment plan, one or two alternate treatment plans, and a minimal plan with your personal expense limitations, you will have a clear picture of your choices.

The Estimate

An estimate is absolutely necessary whenever your dog or cat requires veterinary services. *Leaving your sick pet at a veterinary facility for diagnostic work, surgery, or treatment without receiving an estimate is like leaving a signed, blank check.* Unless you are very familiar with veterinary fees, or can afford to be indifferent to financial shock, an estimate is an absolute must. The estimate you receive should be in writing and it should be accurate. An estimate that includes a range to allow for any "unanticipated problems" is not an estimate at all. A discussion of the unanticipated problems that might arise should be part of the discussion of the treatment plan. How can you make a rational financial decision if the estimate range is between four and eight hundred dollars? The only exception to this is for estimates given for emergencies. These estimates will frequently be given as a range since there is no way to predict the exact treatment plan needed to get through life threatening situations.

There are three types of estimates you might receive, and you should make certain you know which of the three you are being given:

1. The estimated cost, usually given as a range, to get through an immediate, life threatening emergency. This includes treatment for shock, profuse bleeding, respiratory collapse, and other immediate dangers to the continuation of your pet's life.

2. The estimated costs of the diagnostic plan needed to go from a presumptive diagnosis to a final diagnosis. As mentioned earlier, these costs are for laboratory work, x-rays, exploratory surgery, and other diagnostic procedures.

3. The estimated cost for the actual treatment plan once a final diagnosis has been made, including aftercare and recommended medications.

Make certain you receive a copy of any estimate you are given. This copy is important if you decide to get a second opinion. Additionally, having a copy of the original estimate is essential if any conflict develops concerning the total fees charged.

How accurate should your estimate be? When the amount of money you have available to spend for food and shelter for yourself or your family is involved, you don't want an estimate. *You want to know exactly how much it is going to cost.* That figure is available to you if you tell your veterinarian that you are on a tight budget and you can't afford even one dollar more than the estimated amount. If this notation is written on your pet's medical record you can be very certain that the entire staff will carefully avoid spending any of your money without your prior authorization. Under these conditions, if your veterinarian carelessly forgot a couple of items when making your "estimate," there is an excellent chance these items will not even show up on your bill. If they do, they will usually be adjusted off as soon as you remind the receptionist or your veterinarian of your stipulation.

THE BILL

There are three times when you might be presented with a bill or requested to leave money. The first is when you are leaving the facility with your pet after an office visit. The second is when you are leaving your pet at the facility. The receptionist may ask you to leave a deposit. The third is when your pet is discharged from the hospital. Unless you have specifically made arrangements to make payments, you will be expected to pay the bill when it is presented to you. Most veterinarians accept cash, checks, money orders, and major credit cards, such as master card and VISA. Although it might require a credit application, try to establish credit if your veterinarian allows charge accounts. This will allow your veterinarian to send you a monthly statement and you will save credit card interest. Some veterinarians charge interest, but sometimes only after a grace period and sometimes at a rate that is lower than a typical credit card rate.

The bill you receive should be itemized and complete. It should show a breakdown of every item your pet received and the cost for each item. A bill that clumps all, or most, charges under the heading "professional services" is not a satisfactory bill. You have no fees to compare if you later decide a comparison is necessary and you don't know for certain whether other charges, such as charges from an outside laboratory, might show up later. Many veterinarians use computer generated bills. These bills are not only complete, but are an actual medical record of your pet's illness or injury. All itemized bills should be made a permanent part of your pet's medical record and should be kept in a safe place in your home.

When you receive your bill you should check each item and double check to make sure there are no addition errors. Bookkeepers sometimes spend hours trying to reconcile the daily charges with the daily receipts. Many errors are overcharges. When an overcharge is discovered the client's account is, of course, properly adjusted, but many veterinarians do not have bookkeepers and never discover why the charges and receipts seldom add up properly at the end of each day. If you fail to check your bill, it could be your overpayment that is causing the problem.

COST WORKSHEET

          <u>COST</u>

    a. Initial Office Call and Exam Fee: $_____.

PRESUMPTIVE DIAGNOSIS: _____

Diagnostic Plan Expenses:

    a. Lab work needed? $_____.
    b. X-rays needed? $_____.
    c. Anesthesia needed? $_____.
    d. Surgery needed? $_____.
    e. More complete exam needed? $_____.
    f. Miscellaneous needed? $_____.

FINAL DIAGNOSIS: _____

Treatment Plan Expenses:

    a. Treatment needed? $_____.
    b. Surgery needed? $_____.
    c. Hospitalization needed? $_____.
    d. Medication needed? $_____.
    e. Special Diets Needed? $_____.
    f. Follow-up Visits Required? $_____.
    g. Follow-up Lab and X-rays Required? $_____.
    h. Miscellaneous? $_____.

TOTAL ESTIMATED EXPENSES: $_____.

ALTERNATE TREATMENT PLANS:
    PLAN A $_____.
    PLAN B $_____.
    MINIMAL PLAN $_____.

LESS DISCOUNTS OR ADJUSTMENTS: $(_____).

TOTAL: $_____.

YOUR PERSONAL EXPENSE LIMITATION: $_____.

CHAPTER 2:

UNDERSTANDING THE ESTIMATE

A detailed estimate is as important as the estimate itself. If, upon being asked for an estimate, your veterinarian tears off a paper towel, stares off into space for a few seconds, and then writes down a couple of figures and a total, you really don't have much. There are detailed estimate forms available to veterinarians from many sources, and computer generated estimates are being used in many veterinary facilities. *Your copy of a detailed estimate is the only thing that stands between you and an open ended contract in favor of your veterinarian.*

Most estimates combine subtotals into several categories, such as surgery, treatments, hospitalization, laboratory, x-rays, and dispensed medications. There will likely be a few categories in the estimate that will need some clarification, and others that may need to be negotiated. The most likely categories are detailed in the following paragraphs. An estimate is only useful when you understand all the parts.

HOSPITALIZATION CHARGES

Most veterinarians charge a fee for every night your pet spends in the hospital. This usually shows up on the estimate as hospitalization. Since this can become a substantial item, it is important that you find out what you are getting. It is also important to take advantage of proper timing. If, for example, your pet requires minor surgery, try to make an early morning appointment. This allows time for your pet to recover from the anesthetic and be ready to go home the same day, avoiding overnight hospitalization. Since the hospitalization fee is usually added to patient records each morning, the time your pet is discharged from the facility can make a difference in your final bill. If your pet is admitted to the hospital on Monday morning and goes home Tuesday evening you will likely be charged for only one day of hospitalization. If your pet is admitted Monday evening and goes home Wednesday morning you will be charged for two days of hospitalization, even though the number of actual hours spent hospitalized is almost the same in both examples.

$ **TIP:** *Whenever possible, avoid additional hospitalization charges by having your pet discharged from a veterinary facility in the evening instead of the following morning.*

Different veterinary facilities offer different levels of hospitalization. There are some veterinary facilities, mostly in larger cities, that are open 24 hours each day. Even in the middle of the night, a staff, including a veterinarian and veterinary assistants, is present. In these facilities, patients are monitored and body temperatures, pulse rates and respiration rates are taken continually during the night by fully trained personnel. Intravenous fluids and oxygen can be administered 24 hours a day without interruption, and any necessary emergency treatment can be started immediately. If your pet is critically ill or critically injured, he or she should be hospitalized in such a facility. Emergency pet clinics usually offer the same level of care at night, but these are usually only open at night, on weekends, and on holidays, so your pet needs to be moved to a daytime facility each morning.

Those daytime veterinary facilities that are not open 24 hours each day, offer varied levels of hospital care at night. Some have trained night attendants to monitor the patients at night, with a veterinarian on call if an emergency arises. Others have night attendants who make the rounds of hospitalized patients a couple of times each night, but are not required to stay awake all night and are provided sleeping accommodations. *Most daytime veterinary facilities do not have anyone present between closing time at night and opening time the next morning.* In some States, a veterinarian is required to notify their clients, in writing, if there will not be anyone in the facility at night.

If a cost for hospitalization is part of your estimate, you should find out exactly what level is offered in your veterinarian's facility. If your veterinarian informs you that a night attendant is present, you should ask for further information. An experienced attendant checking on the patients every hour or so, taking the temperature of the sick patients, and monitoring the administration of oxygen or intravenous fluids can make a big difference to your pet. An untrained night attendant asleep in a soundproof room is not going to be much help to your pet, even if this allows your veterinarian to indicate that a night attendant is available.

The fact that different veterinarians offer different levels of hospital care at night is cause for both financial and medical concern. If your pet only needs rest and time for recuperation, hospitalization in a facility with a nighttime staff may be too expensive. You can provide rest just as easily at home, and at a greatly reduced cost. If, on the other hand, your dog or cat is recovering from surgery, or is severely ill and requires constant supervision or frequent medication and treatment, you will want him or her hospitalized in a facility with a medical staff that includes a veterinarian on the premises at night, even if this means transferring your pet to such a facility at night and back to your usual veterinarian in the morning.

Unless there are good medical reasons to the contrary, dogs and cats usually do better at home than in a veterinary hospital. Recovery is often faster and expenses are greatly reduced. If necessary, you can supply casual observation by putting your pet next to your own bed at night. While you might not be medically trained, you can certainly provide more observation than your pet would receive if hospitalized in a facility with no one present. Additionally, it is often less expensive to take your pet back to your veterinarian for a recheck and necessary treatment each morning than it is to leave your pet hospitalized.

$ **TIP:** *If your pet requires hospitalization, make certain he or she is in a facility offering constant medical supervision and immediate professional help if needed. If your pet does not require such supervision, he or she will often be better off at home, and your savings of BIG BUCK$ will be considerable.*

LABORATORY AND X-RAY CHARGES

There are two ways your veterinarian can get laboratory work done on your pet's blood. The first is to draw the blood sample and send it out to a commercial laboratory. The report is usually sent back to your veterinarian the next day. The second way is for your veterinarian to invest many thousands of dollars and put an analysis machine in his or her facility and do the blood work in-house. If your veterinarian can do the work in-house, the results are obtained 12 to 24 hours quicker. This is unimportant for routine screening, but very important in acute care situations. The disadvantage is that the operation of the machine requires technical ability and, if doing only a few tests daily, your veterinarian may have to charge more for the tests than a commercial laboratory, running hundreds of tests daily, will charge. If your veterinarian sends the laboratory samples out to a commercial laboratory, try to avoid leaving your pet in the hospital while awaiting laboratory results.

$ **TIP:** *The longer your pet is hospitalized the greater the expense and the greater the chances are that your pet will contract another disease that is unrelated to the initial problem.*

When your veterinarian recommends blood testing you should ask why. Since a full panel of tests may cost between fifty and one hundred dollars, you not only need to know why the tests are being recommended, but also you need to be the one who makes the final decision on running these tests. One reason your veterinarian might give you for recommending blood testing is to determine normal values against which future comparisons can be made. While this is a medically sound reason, you need to decide if such a data base is worth the expense involved. Your own financial ability must be the determining factor.

Another reason for blood testing is to find out if there are any problems that might complicate the use of a general anesthetic. Consider a very routine procedure such as a dental prophylaxis (teeth cleaning) as an example of this use. If your veterinarian recommends that your pet's teeth be cleaned while under a general anesthetic, and recommends a laboratory panel to find out if there are any ongoing disease processes that might complicate the actions of the anesthetic, you have several options available. Your veterinarian is actually asking you to authorize four different procedures. First, you are being asked to authorize the expense of the laboratory work. Second, you are being asked to authorize any treatment necessary if the laboratory results are not normal since there would be no reason to have the laboratory work done if you don't want or can't afford the treatment. Third, you are being asked to authorize the administration of a general anesthetic, and fourth, you are being asked to authorize the cleaning of your pet's teeth.

Your options are more clearly seen if you take the above list and go backwards. You know your pet's teeth to be cleaned and you want the procedure done, so you authorize the cleaning. The general anesthesia has to be given since dogs and cats just don't open wide when asked, so you also authorize the anesthetic. The function of the liver and kidneys is of great concern when considering the use of a general anesthetic, and when the laboratory tests show either of these are not functioning normally, proper treatment may improve the anesthetic risk. Such treatment, however, usually requires hospitalization and can be expensive. This is the medically best way to proceed and, if such treatment falls within your expense limits, you should to authorize the laboratory tests and any necessary treatment. If, on the other hand, such treatment is beyond your economic means, you might be better off having the anesthetic given and your pet's teeth cleaned without the expense of the laboratory work. There is an increased risk, but with severe tartar build-up and gum disease, the risk of the anesthetic is usually less than the risk of doing nothing at all. Once the gums become severely infected the infection can spread and fatally damage internal organs such as the kidneys and the heart.

$ **TIP:** *If your budget is limited, try not to get caught in a financial spiral.*

A financial spiral is created when one medical test or procedure leads to another until you have so much money invested that the decision to spend more money is primarily made to protect the amount already spent. Laboratory testing is a frequent beginning point for the creation of a financial spiral. If one of the tests is abnormal it is likely that a more sophisticated test will be required to aid in the diagnosis. The sophisticated test results may indicate the need for a surgical biopsy or exploratory surgery, either of which may indicate the need for major surgery. When laboratory testing is one of your veterinarian's recommendations, you will need to discuss with your veterinarian all of the possible consequences, including the possibility that an abnormal test result may lead to other tests or other diagnostic procedures instead of leading directly to the final diagnosis.

The most common reasons for recommending laboratory blood testing are to help your veterinarian make a final diagnosis or to monitor an ongoing disease

process. The use of testing in making a final diagnosis was discussed on page 11 and the same principles apply to the use of laboratory results to monitor an ongoing disease process. If you are unable to afford the laboratory work to monitor a disease, you will be impeding your veterinarian's ability to decide if the treatment plan is working, but allowing an experienced veterinarian to follow his or her treatment plan without laboratory monitoring is better than doing nothing about the disease at all.

Find out how your veterinarian charges for laboratory work. If the blood samples are sent to a commercial laboratory, your veterinarian may charge a blood drawing fee plus the laboratory fee, and possibly a handling fee. If this is the case, it is usually less expensive to have a group of tests run all at once. You only have to pay the blood drawing fee once, and most laboratories charge less for a group of tests than they would charge if each test were to be run individually. In contrast, some veterinarians charge a flat fee for each test which includes the laboratory fee, blood drawing fee, and handling fee. Here, just running the tests that are absolutely necessary makes the best financial sense since there is no monetary penalty for running additional tests later.

Whenever you have laboratory work done on your pet, request copies of the results. If you ever require after hours veterinary care, a second opinion, or care from another veterinarian while you are traveling, take your pet's health records, including laboratory results, with you. It is an unnecessary waste of **BIG BUCK$** to spend money for laboratory work during the day with your regular veterinarian, and then spend it again a couple of nights later at an emergency clinic because there is no way you can get the results from your veterinarian after hours.

$ TIP: *Copies of vaccination records, laboratory reports, and medical history can save many dollars if you need a veterinarian while you are traveling or need to go to an emergency facility.*

The primary reason for taking x-rays is to confirm a presumptive diagnosis and, like other diagnostic tools, are frequently a necessary part of the proper medical handling of your pet's injury or illness. If your veterinarian suspects your cat has a broken toe or your dog has arthritic hips, x-rays of the affected parts would allow your veterinarian to make an immediate diagnosis. X-rays, however, can be expensive. If, because of the costs involved, you decide not to have x-rays taken, you may be severely impairing your veterinarian's ability to make a final diagnosis. Broken legs, slipped disks, severe pneumonias, obstructed bowels, severely enlarged hearts, and many other problems will frequently go undiagnosed if x-rays are not taken. The symptoms, however, can still be treated. Medicine existed as a profession long before the invention of the x-ray machine, and it is still being practiced in certain areas of the world without such sophisticated equipment. Recognize that you are making things difficult for your veterinarian, but, like laboratory testing, the decision to have x-rays taken is yours to make.

DISPENSED MEDICATION CHARGES

Veterinarians are the only health care professionals permitted to both prescribe and sell prescrip-

tion drugs. Other health care professionals are required to write prescriptions that are then filled by licensed pharmacists. This is probably because veterinarians in the past compounded and used their own set of drugs, and pharmacists either weren't trained in the use of veterinary drugs or didn't want to stock them.

Today, many drugs used in small animal medicine are either stocked in your local drug store or pharmacy or a human equivalent is available. These drugs can often be purchased at less cost from a drug store or pharmacy than purchasing them from your veterinarian. Drug companies give huge quantity discounts, but very few veterinarians can buy in the quantities necessary to qualify for these discounts. A common drug pricing technique used in veterinary medicine is to mark up the cost of the drug by some factor, and then add a pharmacy or dispensing fee. For example, a name brand antibiotic capsule may cost your veterinarian $1.21 per capsule if purchased in lots of one hundred capsules. If your veterinarian uses a mark up of 100% plus a $5.00 dispensing fee, twenty capsules will cost you $53.40, or $2.67 each. A discount pharmacy, buying thousands or even millions of these capsules simultaneously, can probably dispense the same twenty capsules to you for about half that price. Additionally, the pharmacist may advise you that the same medication is available in generic form for about $0.15 each so, with your veterinarian's permission to use the generic form, the twenty capsules bought at a pharmacy may cost less than ten dollars. In addition to discount drug stores and pharmacies, low cost drugs are available by telephone, through the mail, and at least one large retail chain is considering selling drugs by catalog. If you happen to live near either Canada or Mexico, or travel to either of these countries, you will find that prescription drugs cost as little as one tenth as much as the same drug costs in the United States. Veterinarians write the same prescriptions physicians do, so if you want the opportunity to save **BIG BUCK$** on your pet's bill for dispensed medicine, ask your veterinarian for a prescription and do some comparison shopping. Sometimes, however, you will discover that the veterinary form of a drug is considerably cheaper than the human form.

Some commonly used veterinary medications are available in drug stores without a written prescription. Cortisone creams, antibiotic ointments, digestive aids, and antihistamine preparations are examples of these over-the-counter items. With the costs and pricing formulas involved, your veterinarian may have to charge two to five times the amount you would pay for a tube of ointment or a bottle of Kaopectate® purchased at your local drugstore, and the size container you get at the drugstore will probably be larger.

$ **TIP:** *Always ask your veterinarian for a prescription whenever he or she needs to send home medications for you to give your dog or cat.*

An important rule to follow is to not give any human medications to your pet without a written prescription. You can then take the prescription to your pharmacist who can tell you if a human equivalent exists, if it is available in pediatric strength, or if there is an over-the-counter preparation you can use. Unfortunately, some human medications are very poisonous to dogs and cats. This is especially true with human pain medications.

There are certain diseases that require long term medication. This may be months in certain cases, or for the rest of your pet's life in others. Your veterinarian can order these medications in bulk amounts for you, allowing you to realize considerable savings, even over a discount pharmacy. However, you should still get a written prescription and do some price comparisons. Some veterinarians buy their drugs and supplies from full service drug companies, while others buy most of their drugs and supplies from wholesale mail order catalogs. The base price of the drugs from the full service companies is usually considerably higher than the catalog prices, so if you do need to buy your pet's medications in bulk, get prices from several veterinarians as well as human medication sources.

It is rare today for a veterinarian to refuse to write prescriptions for the medications he or she wants you to give your pet. This is because so many veterinary drugs have human drug equivalents which are available at drug stores or pharmacies. Additionally, such a refusal may be a violation of the restraint of trade laws enforced by the Federal Trade Commission. Even if the medication is absolutely not available in a pharmacy, and even if there is no human equivalent available, if you have a written prescription you can go to another veterinarian whose pricing formulas and drug sources may produce a considerable monetary gain in your favor.

CHAPTER 3:

FINANCES

Once your veterinarian has completed the examination, made a presumptive or final diagnosis, and prepared an estimate, your time with your veterinarian is usually limited. Since veterinarians commonly schedule appointments every fifteen minutes, it is likely that, by the time your veterinarian completes the estimate, other patients may be waiting, an emergency may have arrived, or your veterinarian may be needed by another member of the staff. This is very unfortunate because important financial decisions shouldn't be squeezed into the last few minutes of the office visit. The best way to get the most out of the last few minutes with your veterinarian is to be very prepared for the questions you need to ask and any negotiations that may be necessary. The worksheet given on page 17 is a good way to get organized, but there are some financial decisions you need to make even before using the worksheet.

EXPENSE LIMITS

You need to put a price tag on your pet. If this seems cold and heartless, remember that we put price tags on almost every other expense we make throughout our lives, and veterinary expenses should be no exception. Some people drive very expensive cars; others drive economical ones. Some people live in mansions; others live in small apartments. Some people eat at expensive restaurants; others cook vegetable stew and eat at home. These variations exist because we are not all economically equal. It makes sense, then, to conclude that not everyone can afford the same level of veterinary medicine for their pets. Pet ownership will never be free, and expenses for food, vaccinations, and neutering surgery should be put into every pet owner's budget. It is the large, unexpected expense that you need to protect yourself against. Take, for instance, the horrible possibility that you might someday accidentally run your car over your family's dog or cat. You rush your pet to an emergency clinic and you are told the cost for emergency treatment will be five hundred dollars. Consumed with guilt, you give your consent for treatment and pay the five hundred dollars with the last of the available credit on your credit card. With the proper treatment your pet survives the night and the next morning you take your injured pet to your normal daytime veterinarian. His or her estimate to repair the broken leg and fractured pelvis is seven hundred dollars. You leave a check for two hundred dollars as a deposit without the faintest idea where you will get the remaining five hundred dollars. Four days later, when your dog or cat is ready to go home, your veterinarian's receptionist, pointing at the sign that reads: "*All Fees Must Be Paid In Full When Patients Are Released From The Hospital,*" wants you to pay the remaining balance of five hundred dollars—immediately. This situation can be avoided, and this chapter will tell you how.

There may be a time when you are faced with making difficult financial decisions concerning your pet's medical care. The time to set financial limits, however, is when your pet is healthy, not when you are faced with making emotional decisions during an emergency. During the twenty-five years I practiced small animal veterinary medicine I dealt with thousands of pet owners who unexpectedly found themselves faced with making important medical, emotional, and financial decisions. Very few of these owners had prepared themselves in advance for this difficult process. *Only if you determine your expense limits in advance will you know if you need to begin negotiations to see if you and your veterinarian can work out a plan that will allow you to stay within these limits.*

It may be necessary to predetermine more than one amount. The following are examples of expense limits you might consider:

▶ An amount that you absolutely cannot exceed if payment is required at the time of service and you don't have any means to finance the costs.

▶ An amount you can afford to pay monthly if your veterinarian will allow you to make payments, or if you have outside means to finance the costs, such as a credit card or bank loan.

▶ An amount you will not exceed without getting a second opinion.

By setting these limits in advance you will be able to maintain financial control. By not setting any advance limits, you are taking the chance of giving control to either your emotions or your veterinarian, who has no idea of your financial situation.

ALTERNATE TREATMENT PLANS

Once you have set your expense limitations, you **will know as soon as you receive an estimate if further**

negotiations are necessary. If the estimated total you receive is under your established limits in both the total expense and second opinion categories, you can authorize the treatment plan knowing that you are not risking your financial well being. If, however, the estimated total is above your expense limits, you need to ask about alternate treatment plans.

Consider, for example, a situation when the estimated cost of applying a bone plate to your pet's broken leg is seven hundred and fifty dollars. Depending on the type of fracture, there may be other ways to handle the repair. A bone plate, as recommended in the initial treatment plan, may be the best way, but this is also likely to be the most expensive approach. For a lesser amount, a pin might be inserted into the broken bone allowing enough stability for healing to occur. If the broken ends of the bone are close to each other a cast might suffice, reducing the costs significantly. However, if a cast is used without providing proper stability of the broken bone, healing may eventually take place, but there may be a lack of proper alignment which may cause the leg to lack normal function. While this is not desirable, it may be preferable to economic euthanasia—euthanasia requested solely for economic reasons. The least expensive approach would be to do nothing except treat the pain and try to keep your pet from moving about. There are many dogs and cats roaming around who once had broken legs that were never fixed. Some of these limp and others have permanently useless legs, but they are alive. There are, unfortunately, injuries and diseases that are so severe that euthanasia must be considered, but these are the exceptions and are far less common than you might suspect. Concerning euthanasia, most veterinarians would never consider making such a personal and emotional decision for you, but if you ask about euthanasia during a discussion of your pet's case, your veterinarian will likely give you the information you need to make a decision, either for or against euthanasia, without you having to wonder if you made the right choice.

Another example of an alternate treatment plan concerns a dog or cat with an ear infection. Proper medical protocol would be to give the patient a sedative or anesthetic, completely examine the ear canal, and send a sample of the pus to a laboratory. The laboratory could then grow the infection and run the tests necessary to identify the causing organism and find out which antibiotic is the most effective, at least under laboratory conditions. While waiting for the laboratory results, which might take seven to ten days, your veterinarian would probably prescribe an ear medication for you to use. The only problem with this, besides the fees charged for the office call, sedation or anesthetic, ear examination, ear cleaning, laboratory work, and dispensed medication is that, by the time the laboratory report comes back, there is a good chance that the temporary medication has worked and your pet's ears are no longer infected. In this case, an alternative to the initial treatment plan would be to request that your veterinarian dispense a medication that has proven effective in eliminating other ear infections, and then try this medication before going to the complete plan.

$ **TIP:** *Remember, your veterinarian is going to assume that you want the very best for your pet and is going to recommend the best treatment plan first, and then offer alternate plans if you ask.*

The above alternate approach for the treatment of an ear infection is an example of a money saving technique called: "diagnosis by treatment." A final diagnosis was never made, and antibiotic sensitivity was never determined, but, by using a medication that is usually effective, the ear healed. After the ear healed, hindsight can be used to determine the diagnosis and the proper medication to use, hence the term, "diagnosis by treatment." Unfortunately, diagnosis by treatment isn't very good medicine. It only treats the symptoms and leaves many unanswered questions. For some pet owners, however, it may be the only alternative if they are unable to afford the tests, x-rays, and sophisticated examination techniques necessary to make a final diagnosis, and it is usually preferable to doing nothing. Veterinarians don't like this approach because they are afraid that they may incur liability problems if the condition worsens or proves fatal due to lack of a final diagnosis. If, for financial reasons, you insist on this approach, your veterinarian may wish to reduce his or her liability by asking you to sign a form saying that you are declining the recommended treatment plan. Don't be intimidated by such a request. Your veterinarian is only trying to protect himself or herself, and is not trying to coerce you into approving a treatment plan you cannot afford. Only you know what your financial limitations are and this approach gives your pet a chance to recover.

FINANCIAL ARRANGEMENTS

Before you make any final decisions based on the estimate you have just received, the time has come for a candid discussion, *with your veterinarian*, about finances. The only person in the office that is in a position to help you in this area is your veterinarian, but this may be a problem since he or she probably doesn't want to talk about finances with you. Most books concerning the business of veterinary medicine, and most veterinary financial advisors recommend that veterinarians not discuss financial arrangements—that they assign this job to someone else in the office. The reason is because many veterinarians are uncomfortable talking about money, and are uncomfortable about having to be a firm businessperson instead of a compassionate doctor. For you, however, there are two very important reasons why you should talk directly with your veterinarian about these matters. First, most veterinarians are compassionate and very much want to be able to help you and your pet. Secondly, the veterinarian is usually the one with the authority to make financial decisions. Why talk to a staff member who has been instructed not to lower fees, not to allow deferred payment plans, and to ask for payment either before treatment or when the pet is discharged from the hospital, and no exceptions? That person is going to say no because it is his or her job.

$ **TIP:** *The person most likely to help you make acceptable financial arrangements is your veterinarian.*

Your goal is not to try to find a way to afford your veterinarian's recommended treatment plan, but to have your veterinarian recommend a treatment plan that you can afford. Therefore, the primary purpose for discussing finances with your veterinarian is to find out what he or she can do to bring the cost of the medical treatment to within your financial limits. Your veterinarian can do this by suggesting less expensive treatment plans, offering a monthly payment plan, or allowing discounts. If, during an examination, your veterinarian discovers your pet has a breast tumor, the recommended treatment plan would probably include a chest x-ray, presurgical laboratory screen, general anesthesia, surgical removal of the tumor, an ovariohysterectomy since these tumors are less likely to spread or recur in spayed pets, a biopsy of the tumor, and whatever hospitalization and aftercare that might be required. If the estimated cost for all this exceeds your expense limitations tell your veterinarian immediately that your budget cannot be stretched to accommodate this much expense. After expressing this to your veterinarian, he or she might propose omitting the presurgical blood screen and the tumor biopsy. These omissions would significantly reduce the estimated charges. Additionally, your veterinarian may agree with your suggestion that you make monthly payments. The result of this discussion is that, instead of a large and immediate cash outlay, your veterinarian has agreed to accept monthly payments on a reduced amount. These negotiations may have made the surgery you couldn't afford, affordable. Further reductions in the treatment plan are possible, if necessary, all the way to the removal of a small tumor mass as an out-patient surgery done under a local anesthetic. Each reduction, however, either costs you knowledge or increases the chances for a reoccurrence of the tumor, and must be considered with care.

$ **TIP:** *Like other forms of negotiation, the person who first mentions a dollar amount usually loses. Once you have agreed that a payment plan is an option, ask your veterinarian what is the minimum amount he or she will accept each month.*

If, instead of discussing the financial problem with your veterinarian, you had taken the estimate to the receptionist, he or she would probably ask for a deposit and inform you that it is customary for the bill to be paid in full when your pet is sent home. This is what most receptionists are instructed to do and say. At this time, such implied inflexibility might cause some pet owners to decide to have nothing done, increasing the risk of having the tumor spread. Other owners, unaware of alternate treatment plans or payment plans, might even request euthanasia.

Lastly, after agreeing on a treatment plan and an affordable payment plan, don't fail to ask the receptionist if you qualify for any discounts. Many veterinarians give senior citizen discounts, military discounts, and professional discounts to others in the medical profession. Don't pass up this opportunity to save **BIG BUCK$** simply because you were reluctant to ask if you qualify for any discount.

FINANCIAL PROBLEMS

There are going to be times when even the best intentions don't work out as planned. If you are unable to make a promised payment when due, try to make some payment, even if only a few dollars. Almost all veterinarians have some accounts receivable and send out monthly bills. Regardless of whether this billing is done by computer or by hand, the financial records that are tagged as problems are usually those that had no payments received during the billing period. Even if you are unable to send the amount promised, it is important that you send something each month. If you are unable to send even a small payment, or if you will be unable to send the promised amount for several months, then you should contact the person in charge of billing and explain the situation. A financial record showing some monthly payment received, or including a reasonable explanation, will usually not be turned over to an outside collection agency.

CHAPTER 4:

SECOND OPINIONS

There are two major reasons for obtaining a second opinion. One is to get a second diagnosis and the other is to get one or more alternate, and hopefully less expensive, treatment plans. Since the primary purpose of this book is to present, for your consideration, a collection of money saving ideas, it is not in keeping with that purpose to describe how to obtain the ultimate in veterinary care for your pet, regardless of the cost. In dealing with second opinions, therefore, I am not discussing diagnostics, only treatment plans. I am not discussing veterinary expertise, only expense. If your usual veterinarian says that your pet has a certain problem and it will cost a certain amount of money to have him or her treat the problem, I am assuming your second opinion veterinarian agrees with the diagnosis. Hopefully, your second opinion veterinarian has, based on his or her experience, an alternate treatment plan that will be both successful and less expensive. When you start getting conflicting diagnoses you are probably dealing with a complicated issue involving higher than normal expenses and, if within your budget, you probably should consider a specialist.

$ **TIP:** *If your veterinarian recommends a treatment plan that is going to cost more than ten times what a second opinion will cost, you should get a second opinion. If, for example, the consultation fee for a second veterinarian's opinion is twenty-five dollars, you should get a second opinion if the original estimate is ten times twenty-five dollars, or two hundred fifty dollars.*

Once you have an estimate, a clear understanding of what the estimate represents, and an understanding of your veterinarian's alternate treatment plans and what they cost, you should apply the automatic second opinion limit as outlined above. The "ten times the consultation fee" doesn't have to be a firm rule, and can be increased, decreased, or changed into a specific dollar amount depending on your circumstances. If consultation fees are forty dollars in your area, you might want a second opinion for an estimated cost of less than four hundred dollars, or, if a second opinion fee is ten dollars, you may not want a second opinion until your estimate has exceeded twenty times that amount, or two hundred dollars. Once set, however, it is best not to waver from this limit, even if it involves moving your sick or injured pet from one location to another. You have a considerable amount to gain and very little to lose when you get a second opinion.

The purpose of a second opinion is not to question your veterinarian, but to recognize that all veterinarians are not identical and to take advantage of another doctor's knowledge and experience. There are sometimes many acceptable ways of handling the same problem, and some are going to be more expensive than others. Additionally, some veterinarians are more hesitant than others in offering alternate treatment plans. When you get a second opinion, you are getting twice as much opportunity to become aware of new or different money saving techniques. Second opinions are so effective in lowering medical costs that many human insurance companies require their policyholders to obtain a second opinion before authorizing any expensive procedure, treatment, or surgery.

When seeking a second opinion, there are a few guidelines you might want to follow:

- Consider choosing a veterinarian outside your immediate geographical area. If you have friends or relatives in a different town or nearby city you might ask them for a recommendation.

- Consider choosing a veterinarian likely to be acquainted with your pet's problem. A veterinarian dealing primarily with farm animals might not be familiar with as many ways to treat your dog or cat's problem as a veterinarian dealing exclusively with small animals.

- Consider choosing a veterinarian practicing in a suburban or rural area if your usual veterinarian's practice is in the city. The overhead costs in rural areas are considerably lower than in cities. Veterinary fees are also frequently lower.

- Consider choosing a veterinarian in a multiple veterinarian practice if your usual veterinarian practices alone. There is a good chance your pet will be examined by more than just one doctor, usually at no additional cost, or that there will be a veterinarian in the practice with a special interest in your pet's problem.

Take as much information to your second opinion veterinarian as possible. Some veterinarians will lend you any x-rays taken, and will give you copies of your pet's medical record and any laboratory reports. Others will request that the second opinion veterinarian's office call for such information. No matter how the information is transferred, the important thing is to avoid having the second opinion veterinarian repeat any diagnostic work already done, and for which you have already been billed.

Sometimes your veterinarian will recommend that you see a specialist for a second opinion. Specialists exist today in many aspects of veterinary medicine such as dermatology, emergency medicine, internal medicine, and ophthalmology. These veterinarians are superbly educated and exceptionally experienced in their chosen field. They have had to prove their knowledge to their peers by way of extensive examinations. Specialists can also be very expensive. As mentioned earlier, this is a book on saving money, and not a book on obtaining the very best in veterinary medical care regardless of the cost. To save **BIG BUCK$**, you might consider making a specialist your third choice, after a specialist has been recommended by both your first and second opinion veterinarians.

There is another source for second opinions that you might consider, the veterinary school nearest your location. There are thirty veterinary schools in the United States and Canada. It is very important for these schools to have a variety of cases available in their small animal clinics, for this is the way veterinary students get clinical experience. No student, of course, is put in charge of a case, but working with an experienced veterinarian in a veterinary school setting is a very important part of a veterinary student's education. If you think it might be to your advantage to have your pet seen at a veterinary school, it is likely that you can get some information by telephone (see appendix C). Even though veterinary schools charge fees similar to the fees charged by private practice veterinarians in the area, the financial advantages can be considerable if you consider what you are receiving. A patient with an especially interesting problem may be examined by more than one very experienced veterinarians, possibly veterinarians who are considered experts in their field or speciality, and by many students. Additionally, veterinary schools frequently have sophisticated equipment that is financially unavailable to veterinarians in private practice.

While not really a second opinion, there are books available that describe dog and cat diseases and their treatments. One such book, *CURRENT VETERINARY THERAPY*, is considered the "Bible" for small animal practitioners. This book discusses the causes and treatments of diseases in great detail. Most veterinarians have a current edition of this book in their collection, and most would be happy to allow you to read any sections that apply to your pet's disease. This book, as well as others about the diseases of dogs and cats, might be found in large public libraries. The larger libraries would probably also have the equipment that would allow you to make a copy of the sections that interest you. These books were written for veterinarians and are very technical in nature, but a great amount of information is available, even to someone untrained in medicine. With the aid of a medical dictionary, you could get a good understanding of your pet's disease, how it occurs, what the recommended treatments are, and what the outcome is likely to be. If you want such detailed information ask your veterinarian if he or she has a copy of *CURRENT VETERINARY THERAPY* and will let you read it.

CHAPTER 5:

DON'T LET LITTLE PROBLEMS GROW

Although you may try very hard to prevent injury or illness, there will be instances when your pet is going to get sick or get hurt. The actions you take when you first notice such an illness or injury can make a big difference in how much the problem will eventually cost. To make my explanations easier, I will use the following definitions concerning an injury or illness:

GRADE I: These are injuries or illnesses that should respond to home care. If you know what these injuries or illnesses are, and if you are prepared to administer any necessary treatment, they should not involve any expense other than the cost of medications.

GRADE II: These illnesses or injuries are going to require professional help, but not necessarily immediately. With proper treatment at home, you can safely wait until your veterinarian is available during normal daytime hours. This allows you to avoid paying an emergency fee.

GRADE III: These require immediate professional attention and cannot wait. If your veterinarian is unavailable, you must seek assistance at some emergency facility.

You can save BIG BUCK$ every time you take proper and timely action to keep a grade I condition from becoming a grade II, or a grade II condition from becoming a grade III. Consider vomiting as an example. Simple vomiting in pets can be handled in much the same manner as with a child. You should withhold all food and water to rest the stomach, and use a medication such as Kaopectate®, which is available at any drug store without a written prescription. If the vomiting stops, and it usually will, you have just saved the cost of an office call, examination, treatment, and possibly dispensed medication to use at home. If, instead of taking the above simple steps, you decide to ignore the vomiting, the stomach could become so severely sensitized that simple medication and treatment would no longer be effective, and eventually the vomiting can become so severe as to become life threatening. Now the treatment consists of hospitalization, intravenous fluids to treat the dehydration, medications to desensitize the stomach, and laboratory work. This can cost many hundreds of dollars. What has happened is that the condition progressed from a grade I to a grade II and on to a grade III problem because of lack of action on your part. This lack of prompt action can become very expensive.

Timing can also be important. If, in the above example, the vomiting continues in spite of your immediate attention and action, you are dealing with a grade II or III condition that requires professional help. If this occurs during the daytime, the time to seek help is before your veterinarian closes for the day. Unfortunately, vomiting often starts in the middle of the night, and by the time you find out that the condition is not going to respond to simple treatment you may be facing an emergency call. Try calling your emergency provider for advice and to find out if there is a fee increase after a certain time. If so, and if they advise seeing your pet, try to arrive at the emergency facility before the higher fee goes into effect. If the vomiting starts after midnight it may be possible to wait until your veterinarian's facility opens in the morning, thereby avoiding the emergency fee. All decisions such as these require the use of good sense. If your dog or cat is vomiting repeatedly, is depressed, or begins to show blood flecks in the material vomited, don't stay home and try to treat it yourself. You are dealing with a Grade III condition and your emergency provider must be contacted immediately.

Pet owners need to be able to decide what problems should be seen as an emergency. This is the reason I wrote *An Owner's Guide to Emergency Care for Cats* and *An Owner's Guide to Emergency Care for Dogs*. These books allow pet owners to make informed decisions about whether their pet needs emergency treatment in the middle of the night, or whether the problem can wait until morning. These books also detail many things that pet owners can do at home to keep grade I and grade II problems from becoming grade III problems that require immediate emergency treatment.

CHAPTER 6:

AVOID AFTER HOURS EMERGENCIES

When considering ways to save BIG BUCK$, avoiding after hours emergencies is at or near the top of the list. After hours refers to the periods of time when daytime veterinary facilities are closed, either for the night, the weekend, or a holiday. Many, if not most, emergencies can be avoided, but the fact remains that the waiting rooms of veterinary emergency facilities all over the country are filled with anxious pet owners who never thought it could happen to them. Although most pet owners do their best to keep their pets healthy, pets are still going to get into the street, they are still going to get bitten, poisoned, or injured, and there are still many diseases that are not preventable by vaccinations. This is why so many emergency pet clinics exist and why emergency medicine has become a veterinary speciality.

Although you may never need to go to an emergency facility, you should prepare yourself for such an eventuality. There is a good financial reason for such preparation; some sources of emergency services are more expensive than others. The most common providers of veterinary emergency services are as follows:

TWENTY-FOUR HOUR VETERINARY FACILITIES

These full service veterinary facilities are primarily found in large urban areas. They are always open, and a veterinarian and support staff are always present. While the staff is usually smaller at night, there are enough backup personnel available so life threatening emergencies are never kept waiting. Twenty-four hour veterinary facilities are sometimes less expensive than other types of emergency service providers. Some do not charge an emergency or an after hours fee because these facilities are always open and, therefore, there are no "after hours." An additional advantage is that you are not required to transfer your pet anywhere early the next morning, as happens with emergency facilities that are only open at night.

EMERGENCY PET CLINICS

Typically named emergency pet clinics, these facilities are usually located in a building or shopping center store that is not physically associated with a daytime veterinary hospital or clinic. On weekdays they usually open at 6:00 p.m. and stay open all night, closing around 8:00 a.m. the next morning, and they are usually open all day and all night on weekends and holidays. These clinics provide full emergency services, with a veterinarian and staff present during all open hours, but you are required to transfer your pet back to your daytime veterinarian the next morning or at the end of the weekend or holiday period. Emergency pet clinics save the lives of thousands of pets each year. They are well staffed, well equipped, and are open when you need them most.

However, emergency pet clinics are usually the most expensive providers of emergency care. Many are corporations, with stockholders (frequently limited to veterinarians), presidents, and boards of directors. Like other corporate businesses, decisions are usually based on good business principles and the corporate goal is to make a profit. Emergency clinics typically charge about twice what a daytime veterinarian charges for the initial office call and exam, and some raise their exam fee after a certain time, such as 11:00 p.m. or midnight.

Emergency pet clinics are unique in that the medical records of almost every major case seen will be reviewed by another veterinarian. This includes the diagnosis made, every treatment administered, and the fees charged. The reviewing veterinarian will be the veterinarian you see the next morning. For this reason, the veterinarians at emergency pet clinics are more likely to advise complete diagnostic procedures and less likely to offer alternate treatment plans than your regular veterinarian. This is a type of "defensive medicine" and, of course, adds to the costs of emergency care. Interestingly, a veterinarian in a normal daytime practice is likely to spend an entire career and never have a single diagnosis, treatment, surgical procedure, or fee charged reviewed by another veterinarian acting in a regulatory capacity, unless an official complaint is made by a dissatisfied client. Peer evaluation on a routine basis is nonexistent in veterinary medicine.

REGULAR VETERINARY FACILITY

Many veterinarians will see after hours emergency patients in their own facility, on an on call basis. After hours telephone calls are usually screened by either a night attendant or answering service, and the calls that might involve an emergency are forwarded to the veterinarian on call, either at his or her home or by way of a beeper. Once forwarded, the veterinarian will help the caller decide if their pet needs to be seen immediately or if the problem can wait until morning. If the answering service or night attendant cannot reach the veterinarian on call, they will refer the caller to another veterinarian or an emergency pet clinic. Some veterinarians only take emergency calls until a certain time each evening, such as 11:00 p.m., so if it is important that you reach your veterinarian after hours, try to call early in the evening.

Veterinarians willing to open their facilities in the middle of the night for emergencies usually charge an extra fee for this service. This fee, called an after hours fee or an emergency fee, is similar to the fee charged by an emergency pet clinic. The advantage of taking your pet to your own veterinarian instead of an emergency pet clinic is that you don't have to transfer your pet anywhere in the morning. The obvious disadvantage is that, if your pet is seriously sick or injured and requires hospitalization, there is no doctor immediately available once your veterinarian goes back home.

Some veterinarians have evening hours. Find out if there are any near you and what their open hours are. These veterinarians typically do not charge emergency fees during their evening open hours. This can save you money if your pet's problem is not too severe, but if your pet is severely injured or sick you must find out what happens when the facility closes for the night. If the entire staff goes home for the night, and your pet requires hospitalization, ask the veterinarian to refer you to an emergency facility offering full-time patient monitoring. Sometimes the emergency facility will waive the emergency fee when veterinarians refer patients directly from their facility to the emergency facility. This is especially true for patients of veterinarians who hold stock in the emergency clinic.

Many veterinarians do not take emergency calls after their normal closing time. This is understandable since there are few people who can work all night on an emergency and then function normally in the office the next day. It is important that you know if your veterinarian takes emergency calls, and, if not, you need to find out where your veterinarian refers emergencies. Ask if your veterinarian is a stockholder in an emergency pet clinic, and, if so, ask if any discount is given to patients of veterinarians who are stockholders. You should also find out if your veterinarian charges a full office call and examination fee when you transfer your pet back to him or her when the emergency pet clinic facility closes in the morning. The answers to these questions will allow you to discover the least expensive way to get through an emergency in your geographical location.

Four very effective ways to avoid the expense of after hours emergency services are:

▶ Taking whatever preventative measures are necessary to avoid emergencies.

▶ Having the knowledge necessary know what is an emergency and what can wait until morning.

▶ Making proper use of your veterinarian during normal daytime hours.

▶ Making proper use of emergency information sources.

When I recommend that you avoid after hours emergency services, I do not mean that you shouldn't

go if you have an emergency. You should be aware, however, that many emergencies arriving at a typical emergency facility could have been avoided by following the preventive tips given throughout this book. For example, being hit by a car usually creates a true emergency, but this couldn't happen if your dog or cat was always confined, and is therefore considered avoidable. Cesarian section surgery is an expensive procedure frequently done at emergency facilities, but is completely avoidable if your female dog or cat has been spayed.

Knowing when an emergency exists is your responsibility. When you are uncertain about a particular situation and decide to call an emergency facility to find out if your pet should be seen immediately, you will usually be advised to bring your pet to the facility. There are two reasons for this. The first is because individual pet owners see problems differently. Some owners overstate the severity of the symptoms and some owners understate the symptoms. The advice to come to the emergency facility is given, therefore, because of the possibility the symptoms are being understated and because of the importance of not missing a true emergency. The second reason this advice is given is to avoid the possibility of having a client tell a referring veterinarian that they called the emergency clinic and were told that the situation probably didn't need to be seen that night and to call their regular veterinarian in the morning, when, in the opinion of the referring veterinarian, the problem should have been seen immediately. The opposite advice might be given if you call your own veterinarian in the middle of the night and understate the severity of your pet's problem. In this case you will probably be advised to try to wait until morning.

$ TIP: *If you call an emergency pet clinic for advice, you are probably going to be advised to bring your pet into the clinic—even if the problem you are concerned about is not a true emergency.*

The most expensive way of misusing an emergency clinic, and adding to your cost of veterinary medicine, is to use the emergency clinic as your primary source of veterinary care. Many pet owners either do not have a regular daytime veterinarian, and use an emergency clinic for their normal veterinary needs, or their pet has a problem and they wait until the only available professional help is an emergency clinic. In my experiences with emergency pet clinics, both as a director and as the staff veterinarian, I discovered that many pet owners do not even have a daytime veterinarian. Many pets seen at emergency facilities have problems that could have been handled at a daytime facility for far less cost.

There are sources of emergency information available when your regular veterinarian is not available. One is the availability of poison control centers that are set up to help you find out what specific action to take in case of an accidental poisoning, and another is the emergency clinic itself. Both are just a phone call away.

Since many after hour emergencies concern accidental poisoning, it is important to know about poison control centers. If your pet is exposed to any product that might be poisonous, either by eating or external contact, an immediate call to your nearest poison control center will give you valuable information. They may tell you that the product is not poisonous, saving an expensive trip to an emergency clinic, or that the material is very poisonous and immediate professional help is required. Make certain you have the container so you will have a listing of the active ingredients before calling for information. Poison control center telephone numbers can be found in many telephone books, usually in the white pages. A telephone number for a poison control center in each State is given in appendix A of this book. Additionally, your veterinarian may be able to give you phone numbers for veterinary poison control centers, but you may be charged a fee if you call a 900 telephone number.

$ **TIP:** *The misuse of insecticides is a commonly seen cause of poisoning in cats. Many, if not most, flea preparations used on dogs are poisonous to cats, and can even be fatal. You can save BIG BUCK$ if you read the fine print on all insecticide preparations before using them on your pet.*

When calling an emergency clinic for telephone advice, you may discover that there are times when the staff cannot spend much time on the telephone. This is usually due to case overload. Most times, however, you will get someone willing to listen to you and answer your questions. The person you talk to will seldom be the doctor, but the other staff members of emergency clinics are generally quite knowledgeable. You should remember, however, that because of the difficulty in making a diagnosis over the telephone and the fear of missing a true emergency, most emergency facility staff members are trained to advise you to bring your pet into the facility and not try to wait until morning.

CHAPTER 7:

VACCINATIONS

One sure way to save **BIG BUCK$** is to vaccinate your pet. While vaccinations do not prevent all diseases, protection exists for many severe, communicable diseases. For example, the treatment of a preventable viral disease can include costs such as an office visit, laboratory work, hospitalization, intravenous fluids, injections, and dispensed medications. This can run into many hundreds of dollars with no guarantee your pet will even survive the disease. Sadly, many pet owners believe that their pets are safe from these diseases if they never go out of the house. This is simply not true. Some viruses are airborne and others can be carried into homes on people's shoes and clothing.

$ **TIP:** *By having your pet vaccinated against the preventable diseases for a few dollars, you may save the many hundreds of dollars treatment would cost if your pet contracts the disease.*

There are, however, several different ways to get your dog or cat vaccinated, and some are less expensive than others.

REGULAR VETERINARY OFFICE

The cost of vaccines to your veterinarian is very low. The vaccine used to protect a cat against Feline Panleukopenia (also called Feline Parvovirus, Feline Distemper, or Cat Fever), Feline Viral Rhinotracheitis,

Feline Calcivirus, and Feline Pneumonitis costs your veterinarian about $1.25. Each dose of Feline Leukemia vaccine costs about $2.75. The vaccine to protect dogs against Distemper, Hepatitis, Leptospirosis, Parainfluenza and Parvovirus also costs your veterinarian about $1.25. A dose of rabies vaccine costs your veterinarian about $0.65. The cost to you will vary depending on your geographical location, and even between one veterinarian and another in the same area, but will be significantly greater than the cost of the vaccine. Even considering the markup, the cost of the vaccinations given by your regular veterinarian may be relatively inexpensive when you consider the extras you receive. You get to make an appointment at your convenience so you don't have to stand in line, you get your pet's medical record updated, you get to talk with your veterinarian, you will get a reminder next time the vaccinations are due, and, if you follow the advice I am going to give you, your dog or cat will get a physical exam at no extra charge.

Many of the money saving opportunities discussed in this book exist because there is considerable competition in veterinary medicine today. To discover the level of competition in your locality, check the yellow pages under veterinarians or veterinary hospitals. If each veterinarian or veterinary facility has only a line or two, you can probably assume that there isn't much competition in your area yet, and some of the money saving tips in this book may not be available. If, on the other hand, the yellow pages are full of large advertisements for veterinarians and their facilities, some outlined in red and others containing cute pictures of dogs and cats, you can assume that there are going to be considerable fee variations and money saving opportunities available. Wherever there is competition, veterinarians often offer extra services, lower fees, or both, to keep you as a client. The services may include: free newsletters, vaccination reminders, liberal billing policies, or even preapproved credit cards that you can use for your veterinary bills. Some veterinarians in highly competitive areas advertise monthly specials or place dollar-off coupons in the local newspapers. These veterinarians are usually very willing to negotiate their vaccination fees, as well as other fees, but you have to ask.

While not necessarily associated with competition, many veterinarians include a free physical exam when they vaccinate your pet. The extent of the physical exam will vary from veterinarian to veterinarian. Some veterinarians feel comfortable just asking you how your pet is and then giving your pet a quick, once over exam. Other veterinarians spend considerable time taking a complete history and then conducting a very complete exam. Since an annual physical exam is an important money saving tip, you should ask if your veterinarian's vaccination fee includes a free examination and, if so, find out if it is a complete exam. If you mentally deduct the cost of the exam from the cost of the vaccinations, you may discover that, if your veterinarian includes a complete exam with the vaccinations, he or she is giving the vaccinations almost for free. This free exam policy can also lead to a fee dilemma for your veterinarian that you can sometimes use to your advantage. If you call your veterinarian's office and make an appointment to have the doctor check your pet's ears, and then, during the appointment, you ask your veterinarian to vaccinate your pet, you will probably be presented with a bill that will look something like the following:

OFFICE CALL/EXAM $20.00
VACCINATIONS.......... ....$45.00
DISPENSED MEDICATION ....$ 7.50

TOTAL......... ....$72.50

If, instead of the above, you call and make an appointment to have your pet vaccinated, and then, during that time, you ask your veterinarian to check your pet's ears, there is an excellent chance that your bill will look like this:

VACCINATIONS..... ....$45.00
DISPENSED MEDICATION ....$ 7.50

TOTAL......... ....$52.50

$ **TIP:** *If your dog or cat has a problem that you want examined by your veterinarian, and your pet's vaccinations are due, make an appointment for the vaccinations and ask the veterinarian giving the vaccination to look at the problem. This will often save you the cost of the office call/exam fee since many veterinarians include this fee in the vaccination fee.*

If you have more than one pet, call your veterinarian and negotiate the vaccination fees. Since you will probably be talking to the receptionist, make sure your request for lowered fees is relayed to a veterinarian who can make decisions on matters concerning fees and discounts, usually an owner or partner. If you bring multiple pets to your veterinarian at the same time for vaccinations you can often get a discount, if you ask first.

Don't expect such discounts to be automatically given. You need to request a discount and make the arrangements in advance. If your veterinarian is either unable or unwilling to make such a discount, or if you would rather have a lower cost than free extras, there are some alternate ways to get your pets vaccinated that will save you **BIG BUCK$**.

VACCINATION CLINICS

Vaccination clinics have become very popular with money conscious pet owners. Two kinds of vaccination clinics exist. The first type is held at a certain time and on a certain day each week or month right inside your own veterinarian's hospital or clinic. Your cost to get your dog or cat vaccinated will be greatly reduced, but the extras mentioned earlier, are also greatly reduced. Your pet gets vaccinated, but that is about all. Don't expect the doctor to have time to give your pet a complete physical exam or talk with you at length about your pet's health problems. These clinics are usually run on a first come first served basis, with no appointments accepted, so everyone gets to stand in line. Discounts for multiple pets are seldom given.

The second type of vaccination clinic is the mobile vaccination clinic that rolls around from parking lot to parking lot on certain days for the sole purpose of vaccinating pets. The fees are about the same as a vaccination clinic held in a veterinary hospital or clinic. These mobile clinics seldom keep records and seldom send vaccination reminders. It, therefore, becomes your responsibility to make sure your pet's records are updated and to remember when the next vaccinations are due. Complete physical exams are usually not given and discounts are seldom given to pet owners who bring more than one pet.

There has been a new trend developing in recent years involving vaccination clinics at pet supply stores. The pet business is a multi-billion dollar industry in the United States, and many of those billions are spent on pet supplies and pet foods. To get people to come into their pet supply stores, I have seen ads offering everything from discounted food, free pet supplies, and even free vaccinations given by veterinarians right in the store. In trying to save **BIG BUCK$** on veterinary expenses, nothing makes savings add up faster than getting something free. Check your local newspapers or check with your nearest discount pet supply store for more information.

There are other free services available. Sometimes veterinarians opening a new office will place advertisements offering free examinations, free vaccinations, and free grooming services during their grand opening celebration. You don't have to promise to become a client to take advantage of these opportunities, and to not take advantage of them is like turning down free money being given away by a bank.

DO-IT-YOURSELF KITS

Lastly, if you can't find a source offering free vaccinations, the least expensive manner of vaccinating your pet is to do it yourself. Dog and cat vaccines are available by mail order and even from pharmacies or supermarkets in some locations. This means, however, that you are going to have to properly inject this vaccine into your pet, and you are going to have to risk the possibility of a vaccine reaction. Vaccination reactions are quite rare, but the possibilities do exist. Considering the cost of the vaccine when buying by mail order or from a pharmacy, the possible reactions, the syringe disposal laws, the possibility the vaccine has spoiled because it was not kept cold enough during transit, and the need to stick a needle into your own pet, I would advise taking another approach unless you have some medical training and a very large pet population. Even if you have many pets, you might try to find a veterinarian willing to come to your home and negotiate a reasonable fee for such a service. Remember, a veterinarian can still purchase the vaccines for considerably less than you can, so he or she can still make money while you are saving **BIG BUCK$**.

CHAPTER 8:

SPAYING AND NEUTERING

$ TIP: *If you want to save BIG BUCK$ on your veterinary medical bills over the lifetime of your pet, have your pet spayed or neutered.*

Unless you are a professional breeder, there is absolutely no valid argument against having your dog or cat spayed or neutered. Even the costs involved can be looked upon as an investment if you consider the amount of money that you might save during the life of your pet. Spaying refers to a surgical procedure done to female dogs and cats known medically as an ovariohysterectomy (removal of the ovaries and uterus), and neutering refers to a surgical procedure done to male dogs and cats known medically as a castration (removal of the testicles). Many expensive medical problems are associated with the organs and hormones of the reproductive system, and if these organs and hormones are gone, these problems seldom occur.

There are many false beliefs concerning these two surgical procedures. One is that a female dog or cat makes a better pet if she is allowed to have one litter before being spayed. Another is that having a litter of puppies or kittens born in your home can be a wonderful educational experience for children. These beliefs, over the years, have significantly contributed to the pet overpopulation problem. Female dogs or cats do not make better pets if they have had a litter any more than a woman becomes a better citizen after having a child. As far as education is concerned, a trip to an animal shelter will impress children with the cruel fact that many of these "educational" puppies and kittens eventually become unwanted pets. The overpopulation problem is so severe today that thousands of innocent cats and dogs are being killed each day—estimated to be fifteen million annually—by city pounds and humane societies, because homes for these unwanted pets just cannot be found.

The following list contains examples of expensive problems, seen in either dogs or cats, or both, that can be almost completely avoided by having your female dog or cat spayed:

Birth problems	Cesarean section surgery
Pyometritis	Ovarian Cancer
Breast cancer	Ovarian Cysts
Vaginal tears	Vaginal prolapse
Eclampsia	Uterine Cancer

The false beliefs concerning males include the beliefs that the male cat or dog will miss pleasurable sexual encounters and will get fat if castrated. Breeding is based on instinct, not on pleasure, and since the male frequently has to fight off the other males that have responded to the female, the predominant feeling involved is probably pain. If a neutered male dog or cat no longer spends energy wandering around at night, howling or barking all night, crossing streets and highways, and fighting other males every time a nearby female comes into heat, his calorie use will be reduced. Since a dog or cat becomes fat only by taking in more calories than he burns up each day, you will probably have to reduce the amount of food you feed your pet after he has been neutered, which will save additional **BIG BUCK$**. Neutered males also have considerably fewer accidents with cars and suffer fewer bite wounds. They stay much closer to home since the instinctive actions of responding to a female in heat are eliminated.

Neutered males also have fewer medical problems. Examples seen in either dogs or cats, or both, include:

Bite wounds	Hit by car accidents
Penis injuries	Testicular Cancer
Abscesses	Prostate problems
Perineal hernias	

Once you decide to have your pet either spayed or neutered, there are many different ways to save money:

COMPARISON SHOPPING

The first is known as comparison shopping. This involves telephoning several veterinary facilities and asking how much they charge for the spaying or neutering surgery. Make certain you know the amount of the total. I can't imagine a receptionist or other staff member quoting a fee for the surgery alone and failing to tell you that additional fees are charged for the anesthetic, examination, or hospitalization, but it could conceivably happen. If you get a very low quote, ask for details. A veterinarian's staff receives many of these calls daily, and all concerned should be well aware of what you are asking. When comparison shopping, you may be told that the quoted fee applies only, "if everything is normal." Additional fees are often added to the spaying fees if the patient is in heat, pregnant, or obese. Neutering fees are much higher if your pet has undescended testicles, either one or both, since the abdomen usually has to be opened and explored to find any undescended testicles.

You should be aware that veterinarians tend to charge less for spaying and neutering surgery than for most other surgical procedures. This is primarily because the fees for these surgical procedures are so frequently compared by dog and cat owners. Additionally, many veterinarians try to keep these surgical procedures affordable as a way of contributing their services to help keep the pet population under control. It is unwise to make a judgment on a veterinarian's overall fee structure based on the fees quoted for spaying or neutering surgery.

SPAY AND NEUTER CLINICS

A veterinarian's normal surgery fee for spaying and neutering is sometimes still more than some pet owners can afford. Spay and neuter clinics will frequently offer these surgical procedures at lower prices than your own veterinarian. This is because many of them do nothing else other than spay, neuter, and vaccinate. Some spay and neuter clinics reduce overhead even more by not hospitalizing the surgical patients overnight, so there are little or no nursing costs involved. There is some point, however, when the surgical fee becomes so low that the surgery must either be subsidized by other income such as vaccination income or charitable contributions, or by cutting expenses. Unfortunately, there is no easy way to discover if the facility you have chosen to do the surgery on your pet has elected to reduce expenses to the point where safety is compromised. Both spaying and neutering surgeries require a general anesthetic and, consequently, both involve some risk. The risks, however, can vary from one facility to another, and may not be associated with the fees involved. A well run, well equipped, and well staffed spay and neuter clinic, charging low fees, may have a lower mortality rate than a particular full service facility charging higher fees. The mortality rates for various surgical procedures in different human hospitals are compiled, compared, and published; not just in professional journals, but in some areas these mortality figures are even published in newspapers for everyone to read. Unfortunately, no such data gathering and publishing is done in veterinary medicine. If you are concerned, call your local Better Business Bureau, or other local consumer protection group, to find out if a particular veterinary facility has received any consumer complaints. If the money spent for the surgery is an important factor in your decision to have this surgery done, then a low cost spay and neuter clinic would be a logical choice.

NON-PROFIT ORGANIZATIONS

There are some areas where the local humane society or pound has built a facility and hired a veterinarian to do low cost spays and neuters. These are usually less expensive than your veterinarian or privately owned spay and neuter clinics. This is because most are charitable, non-profit organizations and sometimes receive generous contributions from caring citizens which help subsidize some of the costs involved. These non-profit organizations also pay no taxes. Contact your nearest humane society, city pound, or area animal control office to find out if there is such a low cost facility nearby.

THIRD PARTY ASSISTANCE

There is actually a way to get your pet spayed or neutered free. There are some third party assistance organizations available for pet owners who cannot afford to pay even the lowest fee to have their pet spayed or neutered. Many of these organizations contract with veterinarians who agree to do the surgery at a reduced rate. When an pet owner contacts one of these organizations they are told where to go for the surgery and the organization pays the veterinarian's reduced fee. If any such organization exists in your area you may find the name in your phone book, in newspaper ads, from your humane society or city pound, or from your veterinarian.

POST-SURGICAL COMPLICATIONS

Finally, you must know where to go after hours if something goes wrong because of the neutering surgery. No matter where you chose to have the surgery done, ask this question. If the surgery was done by your regular veterinarian, he or she may be a stockholder in an emergency clinic that will treat surgical complications at no charge or at a reduced charge for stockholder's patients. If the surgery was performed at a spay and neuter clinic, ask where you should go because some of these have made arrangements with other veterinarians in the area to see any surgical complications at a reduced fee. This is especially important since many spay and neuter clinics are only open for short periods daily, and are almost always closed at night.

CHAPTER 9:

MONEY SAVING HEALTH TIPS

During the years I practiced small animal veterinary medicine I realized that a few problems kept recurring. Additionally, I noticed that many of these problems could be avoided by simple preventive actions taken by dog and cat owners. I have compiled these problems and preventive actions into the followings lists. Many of these may seem overly obvious, and others may seem so unlikely to occur that it is easy to believe the situation could never happen to your pet. I can assure you, however, that all of the following situations have occurred frequently enough to earn a place on this list. The following health care tips can save you many dollars, some can save you many hundreds of dollars, and some can even save your pet's life. The first group of tips listed below apply equally to dogs and cats; the other tips, specific to either dogs or cats, are listed last.

TIPS FOR BOTH DOGS AND CATS

1. Keep all fishing tackle in a tightly closed container. Dogs and cats love to play with hooks and lures and sometimes catch themselves.

2. Neither dogs nor cats require cow's milk and usually cannot properly digest it. Even a small amount of cow's milk can have a strong laxative effect, and a larger amount can cause severe diarrhea.

3. Kittens, puppies, and occasionally older cats and dogs will sometimes entertain themselves by chewing on elec-

tric wires. If they chew through the insulation they can receive a severe shock, severe burns to the mouth, and internal injuries that can even be fatal. Make sure you keep all wires out of your pet's reach until he or she has passed the chewing stage.

4. If you have a long haired pet, keep the hair growing around the rectum clipped short. This will help prevent the severely painful condition known as "fecal plug" that occurs when bowel movement is caught in the hair and held against the skin.

5. Never leave your dog or cat unattended in a motor vehicle. Even on cool days the temperature inside a closed car can rise to dangerous levels in a very short time, especially if the vehicle is parked in the sun.

6. While pets and children usually go well together, remember the same does not hold true for pets and children's toys. Small toys are sometimes easily swallowed by dogs and cats and can cause an intestinal blockage. Keep small toys and other small objects away from your pet.

7. Brush your pet's teeth. If the tartar (the dark stuff that sticks to the surface of the tooth) becomes too thick to brush off, have the tartar removed professionally. Tartar accumulation can lead to gum disease, and gum disease can lead to tooth loss, abscessed teeth, and even diseases of the internal organs such as the heart and kidneys.

8. Know if any of your house plants are poisonous to your pets. If so, keep them away from your dog or cat, especially when they are young and have a tendency to chew everything within reach.

9. Proper flea control is necessary to avoid the severe anemias and expensive skin problems caused by flea infestations. Flea control will also help control a type of tapeworm commonly seen in dogs and cats.

10. Many dogs and cats will drink from the toilet bowl. Keep this in mind when you use toilet bowl cleaners. Many of these are toxic and can cause severe chemical burns to the mouth and throat. Keep the lid to the toilet bowl closed whenever you are using these products.

11. Do not use human medications on your pets. Some popular human pain medications are poisonous to dogs and cats. When in doubt, call your veterinarian.

12. Keep all poisons in places completely inaccessible to your pet.

13. On hot, sunny days both dogs and cats will frequently sleep under the car for shade. If you have pets, blow your horn before starting and moving your car.

14. Children will occasionally put rubber bands around their pet's neck, leg, or tail. Be very alert for this because the pressure of the rubber band can cause a severe and painful injury. The band itself is frequently hidden by your pet's hair or the subsequent swelling of the body part involved. A similar problem occurs when collars are put on young, rapidly growing pets. Collars on young pets must be checked for tightness every day.

15. Anti-freeze preparations containing ethylene glycol are deadly poisons. Unfortunately, these preparations have a sweet taste that dogs and cats find attractive. Keep all

anti-freeze containers closed and in a safe place. If you drain this material from your car's radiator, remember to dispose of it safely, and clean up any spills. Fatal amounts are measured in teaspoons.

16. Simple, uncomplicated constipation is almost never a problem in dogs and cats. Any straining, as if your pet were trying to have a bowel movement, should be considered serious and your pet should be taken to your veterinarian for a diagnosis. Don't use a laxative unless your veterinarians recommends it.

TIPS SPECIFICALLY FOR DOGS

1. If you use a chain collar on your dog, keep a pair of bolt cutters in an obvious place known to all family members. It is impossible to imagine the damage your dog can do to itself if the collar becomes stuck in its mouth, or if its leg gets stuck in the collar, or if another dog gets a leg stuck in the collar while playing. Once a dog panics, there is often no way to get the collar unstuck other than by cutting the collar with bolt cutters. Death by strangulation can occur if you can't quickly find bolt cutters.

2. Keep your dog confined to a yard or on a leash. Dogs that are confined very seldom get hit by cars. Dogs that have access to roads usually have a medical history that is both extensive and expensive, and they have a greatly shortened life expectancy.

3. If you must keep your dog tied, be certain the rope is short enough so your dog cannot get tangled, or jump part way over a fence and get hung. Additionally, if you tie your dog inside the open bed of a truck, may sure that the

leash is short enough to make it impossible for your dog to get over the side or off the back and get dragged. This is a commonly seen, frequently fatal, accident in States that have laws requiring dogs riding in any open truck be tied.

4. Keep a bottle of ipecac syrup in your emergency kit for dogs, and make sure you tell your veterinarian you have the ipecac if you suspect your dog has been poisoned. Since vomiting is not indicated in the case of certain poisons and because ipecac syrup is a severe stomach irritant, don't use it to make your dog vomit unless your veterinarian tells you to.

5. If you live in an area having grass seeds or burrs, keep your dog's feet shaved, especially in between the pads and the toes, during the season when these seeds and burrs are present. This will help prevent the severe mechanical damage or abscesses these seeds or burrs can cause.

6. Proper tick control is necessary to prevent Lyme disease and can also help prevent a type of paralysis caused by tick bites.

7. If you have a dog and a swimming pool, you must teach your dog where the steps are located. You can do this by putting your dog in the pool and then providing enough guidance to allow your dog to find the shallow end and the steps. A couple of lessons will go a long way toward avoiding an accidental drowning in case your dog ever falls in. If you have an epileptic dog and a swimming pool, make certain your dog has no access to the pool when adults are not present. A dog having a seizure can drown if he or she is in the pool, or falls into the pool, when the seizure starts.

8. Get some veterinary tranquilizers from your veterinarian if your dog reacts violently to thunder, fireworks, gunshots during hunting season, or other loud noises. Give the medication whenever you suspect these types of noise might occur. A severely panicked dog can jump right through a glass window.

9. Snail poisons are almost as deadly to dogs as they are to snails, and dogs seem to love the taste of this poison. If you have both snails and a dog, find a way to control the snails without harming your dog. The boxes of this poison are clearly marked, but the incredible danger cannot properly be put into words. Your dog doesn't have to eat very much to become severely poisoned.

10. Don't feed your dog bones. There are three areas in the body where they can get stuck and require expensive treatment, or even surgery, to remove. Bones can get stuck in the mouth or throat, in the stomach or small intestine, or the bones can be ground into pieces small enough to pass into the large intestine where they can be turned into a mass very similar to hardened concrete. This mass is usually too big and too painful to pass from the body naturally. Professional assistance, sometimes including sedation or anesthesia, is required to remove this mass of bone chips from the rectum.

11. To help avoid bloat, your dog should receive frequent small meals instead of just one large meal daily. Avoiding heavy exercise and the ingestion of large quantities of water shortly after eating will also help.

12. Keep your dog's toenails at the proper length either by cutting or filing them. This is especially important for

small dogs that are usually kept indoors. Broken and ingrown toenails seldom occur if the nails are kept short.

13. If you cut your dog's toenails and accidentally get one bleeding, a styptic pencil used to stop the bleeding of a razor nick will often work to stop the toenail bleeding. There may be some stinging so don't get bitten.

TIPS SPECIFICALLY FOR CATS

1. If you need to put a collar on your cat, make sure it has some means of breaking away if it gets caught. This also applies to flea collars if you use them.

2. Make sure you keep all sewing materials away from your cat. Needles and thread make wonderful playthings until the needle is swallowed.

3. Containers of bacon grease are very appealing to cats. Eating bacon grease, however, can cause a severe bloody diarrhea.

4. A pillow case makes a good emergency carrier and will make sure your cat doesn't run out into the road when being transported.

5. If you notice your cat straining in the kitty box and only passing small amounts of urine, your cat may have a bladder infection. An additional symptom is the presence of small amounts of blood in the urine. Early detection of a bladder infection is especially important for male cats since it might be associated with feline urological syndrome. An examination, urinalysis, and treatment at this stage may help avoid a complete urinary tract blockage.

6. Feed your cats, especially male cats, a food that has been prepared to help avoid feline urological syndrome by reducing the magnesium content.

7. Cats love to sleep in warm places on cool days. This includes your car's radiator and engine. You would not believe the amount of damage a fan belt can do to your cat before you can turn off the engine. Try to develop the habit of honking your car's horn before starting or moving your car.

CHAPTER 10:

THINGS TO DO AT HOME

There are times when you can be your own veterinary medical provider. You don't have to get professional assistance every time your dog or cat gets sick or injured. To save **BIG BUCK$**, you have to avoid going to your veterinarian whenever possible. However, it is essential that you know *when* to treat your pet at home, and *when* to take your pet to your veterinarian. As previously discussed, it is financially imperative that you avoid allowing a grade one problem to progress to a grade two or a grade three problem by attempting home treatment at the wrong time. Some pet owners are very knowledgeable about medicine and feel comfortable treating their pets at home. Others prefer to have their pets examined professionally at the first sign of illness or injury. Those pet owners in the first category generally spend less money on their veterinary bills than those in the second category.

$ **TIP:** *As a pet owner's knowledge of veterinary medicine, first-aid, and emergency care increases, the number of trips they make to their veterinarian decreases. Knowledge is one of the keys for saving BIG BUCK$.*

BOOKS AND MANUALS

The actions you take when your pet gets sick or injured depend on how much you know about sickness and injury. A pet owner who knows almost nothing about veterinary medicine will usually either over or under react. An overreaction will frequently be too expensive, and an under reaction may put your pet's live in jeopardy. The first step in gaining the knowledge necessary to make the proper decisions is to start a library at home. Books, magazines, and pamphlets, each costing less than the amount most veterinarians charge for an office visit, can frequently save hundreds of dollars in veterinary fees. My books, *An Owner's Guide to Emergency Care for Cats* and *An Owner's Guide to Emergency Care for Dogs*, cover the information you need in case of an emergency. Many other books are available, either in bookstores or in your nearest library, that cover general health care for dogs and cats. Your veterinarian usually has several guides to health care available, and these are usually free. These guides are published by manufacturers of pet products and foods, and many contain coupons for discounts or free merchandise. Make it a point to visit your veterinarian from time to time just to ask for free literature or product information.

TELEPHONE ADVICE

Some of the knowledge needed to make decisions concerning your pet's health problems can be obtained by using your telephone. As mentioned earlier, by calling a poison control center in cases of suspected poisoning you can sometimes save a trip to your veterinarian or emergency facility. The telephone can also be used to obtain advice and get information from several other sources, such as your own veterinarian, an emergency clinic, or breeders in your area. There are, however, some problems associated with relying solely on telephone information when making important medical decisions. These are discussed in the following paragraphs.

Your Own Veterinarian's Staff

Telephones in veterinary offices usually ring constantly. Some are calls from pet owners needing to make an appointment, others are from people doing comparison shopping, and still others are from clients checking on the progress of hospitalized patients. Many calls, however, are calls made by pet owners to ask questions and gain information. When your pet is sick or injured, the answers to your questions become increasingly important to your pet's well being. Because of this importance, you must consider the source of the answers to your questions. *The only staff members qualified to give advice dealing with sickness or injury over the phone are the veterinarians.* This is because they know the proper questions to ask to differentiate between simple, uncomplicated situations and life threatening situations sharing the same set of symptoms. Unfortunately, most veterinarians either can't or won't talk to everyone who calls on the phone. One reason for this is that veterinarians do not want to take time away from the clients and patients already in their facility. Another reason is that many veterinarians want the patient record when they discuss patients over the telephone, either to make notes during the phone conversation or to help jog their memory about your pet's medical history. Even if they can't talk directly with you, many veterinarians will answer questions relayed to them by a staff member. For this reason, the more organized you are, the more likely you are of getting an answer to your questions from your veterinarian.

When calling a veterinary facility for medical advice, give whoever answers the phone your name, phone number, and short history of your pet's prob-

lem. This information should include your pet's age, sex, temperature, and symptoms. Then ask the person answering the phone to please ask the doctor for his or her advice, and suggest that, if the doctor is busy, you would be willing to stay on the phone or ask that the doctor return your call when convenient. Many veterinarians reserve time during each day to return their client's telephone calls. To do so is in your veterinarian's best interest since your dog or cat's problem may need professional attention, which is what he or she does for a living. It is also in your best interest because the problem may not require professional attention, saving you both time and money.

By taking a positive approach and requesting that the question be presented to the veterinarian personally, you are avoiding many possible communication problems. Over the years I have overheard high school volunteer workers giving specific and incorrect health care advice to unsuspecting pet owners with so much confidence the caller could easily believe he or she was talking with an experienced veterinarian. I have also heard inexperienced staff members telling a client that they should bring their pet to the hospital immediately, when the situation required no medical treatment whatsoever. Some veterinary facilities have phones all over the place and the entire staff, including kennel and janitorial personnel, are instructed to answer the phone whenever it rings more than just a couple of times. If you are lucky, an inexperienced, or medically untrained, person may put you on hold; if you are unlucky, the person you are talking to may give you some very faulty advice.

Veterinarians do not want you to bring your pet to their facility, or to spend money with them, when it

is not necessary. Most accomplish this by using personable, compassionate, and knowledgeable receptionists who screen calls, answer questions, and relay questions to the veterinarians whenever necessary. If, when calling a veterinary facility for information and advice, you do not talk to someone like this, and if you are completely put off by being told that the only way they can help is if you bring your pet in for an examination, you might call a second facility and compare how you are treated. Veterinarians today are more concerned with good client relationships than with the fact that they may be giving out free advice. Many years ago, veterinarians were advised by business consultants to instruct their staff that the only purpose of a phone in a veterinary facility is to make appointments, and any other use is giving away income. In the highly competitive world of veterinary medicine today, being treated like this may be an indication that your veterinarian is either unaware of his staff's telephone manners, or that your veterinarian may have an attitude problem that could possibly carry through into other areas.

$ **TIP:** *When you are on the phone to a veterinary facility, and if you are not already a client, you are a prospective new client to that practice if you are treated exceptionally well. If you are already a client, you are a prospective new client to another practice if you are treated rudely or abruptly.*

Emergency Facility Staff

Emergency clinics usually need to handle telephone calls differently. These emergency facilities exist for the sole purpose of saving the lives of pets, primarily when your own veterinarian is unable or unwilling to see and treat patients. Emergency clinic staffs usually don't have time to care about bedside manner and they do not want to establish a long term, warm, friendly relationship with you. They don't want you to send your neighbors, relatives, and friends to them with a glowing recommendation; they just want to be ready and available when they are needed. The doctors and technicians working in a typical emergency facility are among the most compassionate to be found in veterinary medicine. This compassion, however, may cause them to be seem abrupt, since they may worry more about their patient's health than they worry about the pet owner's feelings.

When calling an emergency facility for advice on a medical problem, the information they give you will frequently depend on their case load. If the facility is not busy, you may get more information than you wanted or anticipated receiving. If the facility is busy, they will probably tell you that you are the only one who can decide if your pet needs to be seen as an emergency, and, if you think your pet needs to be seen, you should bring your dog or cat into the facility. Additionally, you may be told the waiting period, if the problem is not life threatening, and the fees you are likely to be charged. While the staff may want to spend more time answering your questions, it is difficult to imagine a veterinary assistant or veterinarian being able to talk to you at length about your pet when the patient they are treating just stopped breathing. The staff of emergency pet clinics operate in the same manner as the doctors and nurses in a human hospital emergency room, and not as trained dispatchers or paramedics answering 911 emergency calls.

Breeders

Breeders of purebred dogs and cats are usually very knowledgeable about their specific breed. This knowledge includes information about medical problems commonly seen in their breed, such as eye problems in collies, hip problems in German shepherds, or bowel problems in manx cats. Many breeders are willing to share this specialized knowledge, and can be an excellent source for second opinion veterinarians who are very experienced with these particular problems. Some breeders and owners have organized clubs that meet from time to time, and sometimes have guest veterinarians as speakers. While you must share the question and answer period with everyone else, you can anticipate getting your questions answered without incurring the expense of an office visit.

PREVENTIVE MEASURES

While considering things that you can do at home, you can save a great deal of money by routinely brushing your pet's teeth. Severe tartar accumulation and associated gum problems require veterinary treatment and can make up a significant amount of the expense of owning an older pet. The bad breath associated with tartar buildup is only a symptom. As tartar accumulates on the surface of the teeth, it pushes the gum away from the teeth allowing pockets to form where bacteria can grow. It is the bacteria and associated infection of the gums that causes most of the bad breath. If the tartar is not removed and the pockets of infection treated, secondary diseases can occur, such as pyorrhea and associated tooth loss, heart disease, and kidney disease. While tartar buildup can occur at any age, the severe secondary problems are usually seen in older dogs and cats. Ask your veterinarian for dental hygiene advice, and have your veterinarian examine your dog or cat's teeth at every opportunity.

A very important thing to do at home is to routinely examine your pet. In order to tell if an abnormal condition exists, you need to know what is normal. I don't believe you need a trained eye to differentiate between normal and abnormal, if your eye frequently sees the normal through all the stages of your pet's life. Start when your pet is young and routinely look closely at him or her, paying special attention to the following:

Eyes	Inside of Mouth
Ears	Hair and Skin
Teeth	Rectal Area
Abdomen and Breasts	Reproductive Organs
Feet, Nails, and Pads	Tail

Nail care is an important treatment that most pet owners can do at home. Torn toenails are commonly seen when a pet's toenails are abnormally long. Most dogs and cats keep their nails at the right length by running and playing on hard surfaces. Additionally, cats climb trees, climb up walls, and use a scratching post to keep their nails at the proper length. Older pets, and pets who stay in the house most of the time, sometimes need help to keep their nails short since they do not have the necessary frequent contact with hard surfaces. The best way for you to help is by filing the nails instead of cutting them. This avoids the possibility of cutting a nail too short and causing it to bleed. Start when your pet is young and the degree of difficulty will be greatly reduced. Some pets become very sensitive about having their feet and nails touched. In these cases, you may have to wrap your cat in a heavy towel and then pull out one leg at a time, or put a muzzle on your dog. It is usually worth the effort to do this at home if possible. It can be very expensive to have your pet's nails trimmed at a veterinary facility if sedation is required.

Bathing and grooming are two more things that you can do in your home. With cats, it is extremely important to know exactly which bathing products can be safely used. Many insecticidal shampoos are for dogs only, and using such a shampoo on your cat can even be fatal. Start bathing your cat at an early age. The easiest way is to place your cat in a sink or tub of water that is about room temperature, and avoid splashing water on your cat. Most cats tolerate water as long as it does not get into their face, eyes, or ears. Dogs can be put into the bathtub or shower, or you can even use the garden hose on warm days. Most dogs like water, but you should avoid squirting water directly into your dog's face.

Pet owners should have an emergency kit in their home for their pets. After thousands of late night telephone conversations with distressed pet owners, I compiled a list of the medical items I would have wanted in each pet owner's home in case of an emergency. This list is on the next page. Sometimes the recommendation to either pay for an emergency call or wait until morning is based on something as simple as your pet's body temperature, but you need a thermometer. These emergency kits can be purchased directly from my company, or can be made from components purchased from a drug store or pharmacy. These kits will also give you the opportunity to save **BIG BUCK$** by putting into your home the supplies necessary to treat grade I problems, and temporarily treat grade II problems until your veterinarian is available, thereby avoiding after hours emergency fees. Each kit should contain the following items:

BASIC EMERGENCY KIT

ADHESIVE TAPE ROLLS
COTTON BALLS
COTTON SWABS
EMERY BOARD OR NAIL FILE
EYE IRRIGATING DROPS (STERILE)
FEEDING/MEDICATING SYRINGE
GAUZE PADS (STERILE)
GAUZE ROLLS
GAUZE SCRUB PADS (NON-STERILE)
GERMICIDAL SCRUB
    (Such as Complexed Iodine Scrub)
GERMICIDAL SOLUTION
    (Such as Complexed Iodine Solution)
GLOVES (LATEX OR PLASTIC)
HEMOSTATIC FORCEPS
IPECAC SYRUP
KAOLIN-PECTIN SUSPENSION
LEASH or HARNESS
LUBRICANT (STERILE)
MUZZLE (DOGS ONLY)
NON-STICK WOUND PADS (STERILE)
PENLIGHT OR SMALL FLASHLIGHT
SCISSORS
SPLINTER FORCEPS
STETHOSCOPE
THERMOMETER (RECTAL) AND CASE
TOURNIQUET
WATERPROOF PAD
PLASTIC CARRYING BOX

CHAPTER 11:

OTHER BUSINESSES

GROOMERS

Veterinarians sometimes offer grooming services in their hospital or clinic facility. Some veterinarians do this by hiring a groomer, while others lease space to a groomer, who then acts independently. Most groomers are very observant and often discover medical problems in the pets they are grooming, such as infected ears, small tumors, infected gums, or tartar build-up on your pet's teeth. A groomer working in his or her own facility can only bring these problems to your attention, but a groomer working in a veterinary facility will usually ask the veterinarian to look at the problem and give his or her advice on what should be done. Since you didn't ask to have the veterinarian examine your pet, most veterinarians do not charge for whatever advice they give. In effect, you are getting a free mini-examination. When you pick up your pet, the receptionist or groomer will tell you that an abnormal condition exists, that the doctor looked at it, and that the doctor recommended that you either watch the problem closely, or make an appointment for a more complete exam. Since the groomer will usually find abnormal conditions at an early stage, this mini-examination can be very useful in avoiding an early problem from becoming worse.

$ **TIP:** *If the cost of grooming is approximately the same, it may save you money if you go to a groomer working in a veterinary facility.*

BOARDING KENNELS

Some veterinarians offer boarding services, and some even have separate facilities for boarding and hospitalization. If your pet requires daily medication or has a medical problem, and you want your pet boarded where medical supervision is available, choose a veterinary facility. However, if you have a healthy pet who is completely vaccinated, a boarding kennel, accepting only healthy pets, has an advantage over a veterinary hospital which accepts both healthy pets for boarding and sick pets for hospitalization. Isolation of sick pets from healthy ones is almost impossible if both are kept in the same physical facility or share the same staff.

PET SITTERS

The best solution to the boarding problem, especially if you have more than one pet, is to have someone come to your house once or twice daily to care for your pets while you are away. This is not only safer from a contagious disease standpoint, but often less expensive than a boarding kennel or veterinary hospital. Some areas have businesses offering bonded and experienced professional pet sitters who come to your house. Professional pet sitting is a rapidly growing business.

EXTERMINATORS

There are certain areas of the country where fleas are a major problem. Fleas are not only dangerous from a medical point of view, but they can be extremely expensive from a pet owner's point of view. Flea allergies are real, and during the height of the flea season many pet owners are forced to get medical help for their pets to control the incessant scratching, hair loss, and skin infections that accompany flea infestations. Having to pay for medicated baths, injections, dispensed medications, and flea control products every four to six weeks can generate horrendous medical bills. Fleas are also the carriers of the larval form of a very common tapeworm. Without fleas, your pet will not be exposed to that type of tapeworm and will not need expensive tapewormings. Additionally, fleas can ingest enough blood to cause your pet to become severely anemic. In very small, or very young, pets this loss of blood can be fatal. Treatment of severe flea anemia requires hospitalization, blood transfusions, intravenous fluids, injections of vitamins and minerals, and even oxygen therapy in the most severe cases. You can save **BIG BUCK$** by getting rid of the fleas in your pet's environment, and the business most likely to help you do this is an exterminating company.

$ **TIP:** *The addition of a professional exterminator to your total flea control program can more than pay for itself in veterinary fee savings.*

CHAPTER 12:

OTHER SUPPLIERS

PET SUPPLIES

Many veterinarians have become merchandisers of pet supplies. This allows a pet owner to shop for pet supplies and pet food while at their veterinarian's facility. While this may save time, it seldom saves money. Discount pet stores and discount warehouse operations can buy pet supplies in huge quantities. The discounts they receive allow them to sell at prices frequently below what your veterinarian has to pay for the items at the wholesale level. As with so many things, you have to pay extra for convenience. If you are willing to shop around and check your newspaper for advertised specials, you can save some **BIG BUCK$**.

Farm animal feed stores frequently supply foods, medications, and supplies for dogs and cats. Prices at these stores are usually considerably less than what your veterinarian charges for the same or similar items. Make certain that any medication you purchase is compounded for small animals, not for farm animals. Any container should be clearly marked that the medication is for dogs or cats. Clerks at these and other similar stores are not pharmacists. You should check with your veterinarian before using any over-the-counter medications.

Many pet stores and farm animal supply stores offer newspapers, newsletters, and brochures that contain dollars off coupons for pet supplies. They also contain advertisements from stores offering supplies at loss leader prices, and sometimes even free, as an enticement to get you into their stores.

Catalogs are available which contain almost every imaginable item you might want for your dog or cat. These catalogs are usually free and advertise their existence in many dog and cat magazines.

Pet foods are a major part of the expense of owning a pet. It is not necessary to feed the most expensive brands, nor is it wise to feed the cheapest. In this age of enlightened nutritional awareness, dog and cat food manufacturers are very aware of the nutritional value of their foods, and are very aware that consumers are not going to buy pet foods lacking nutritional value.

DOG FOODS

Good nutrition can be obtained from many of the medium priced dog foods produced by the name brand companies. The expensive foods costing $35.00 or so for forty pounds—almost $1.00 per pound if you have to pay tax—are excellent foods, but forty pounds of a very nutritious food can cost about one-third of that price when purchased at a discount supermarket, discount pet store, or discount feed store. The question is not whether one is better than the other, but whether the expensive food is almost three times better than the others. The nutritional difference between the most expensive and middle priced food is nowhere near the price differential. The very inexpensive dog foods are mostly indigestible bulk. Dogs that eat these foods must eat large quantities to fulfill their nutritional needs, and you will probably need a truck to haul away the backyard cleanings.

It is important to recognize that the nutritional needs of growing puppies, mature dogs, and old dogs are very different. Most dog food manufacturers also recognize this and produce foods meeting the nutritional requirements of dogs of different ages. Discuss nutrition with your veterinarian. If your veterinarian recommends a very expensive premium dog food that he or she sells, explain that your budget cannot handle that much expense and ask for a second choice. Remember, because the foods must be paid for and stored in valuable hospital or clinic space, most veterinarians mark-up the foods they sell by 30% or more. Very few veterinarians will refuse to see your pet as a patient because you cannot afford a particular brand of food.

CAT FOODS

Cats are not finicky eaters. They do not require the expensive little cans of food we so often see advertised. Dry foods have the same nutritional value, are less likely to spoil, and are considerably less expensive. In over twenty-five years of caring for the medical needs of cats I have never encountered an otherwise healthy cat who wouldn't eventually eat dry food—with great enthusiasm—once he or she got hungry enough. If, however, you have an older or very overweight cat who only eats canned food, you should consult with your veterinarian if your cat does not start eating the dry food you are offering within 24 hours.

Male cats have special nutritional needs. Many manufacturers of cat food now recognize the role magnesium plays in plugged urinary tracts of male cats. Foods that are low in the element magnesium greatly reduce the incidence of these urinary tract blockages. Since the treatment of a male cat with his urethra (the tube leading from the urinary bladder through the penis to the outside) plugged can cost many hundreds of dollars, I recommend feeding male cats only those products clearly labeled that they are low in magnesium, or prepared to reduce urinary problems, or some similar words. By using these foods you will greatly decrease the chances of your male cat getting a plugged urethra.

SPECIAL DIETS

If your dog or cat has a disease and your veterinarian advises a special diet as part of the treatment, ask your veterinarian if there is a recipe for a homemade equivalent. These diets, some of which can only be purchased through your veterinarian, are very expensive. They frequently cost between $1.25 and $1.50 per pound. There is often an equivalent that you can make at home. If you have the time to do the preparation, you can buy the ingredients and make a substitute diet for considerably less that the cost of the special diet. These life saving diets are based on the same dietary recommendations our physicians would make if we had a similar condition. If, for example, your dog has a heart problem and your veterinarian recommends a special diet with a reduced sodium content, you can buy one of many books dealing with restricted sodium diets for people with heart disease. These books usually contain lists of foods that are low in sodium. Some veterinary medical books, such as *Current Veterinary Therapy*, give recipes for some special diet equivalents.

CHAPTER 13:

MISCELLANEOUS TIPS

Veterinary medical expenses are not generally deductible on your income tax forms. However, many clients have told me that they do deduct some or all of the expenses involved in owning a pet, including veterinary expenses, pet food costs, pet supply costs, and even grooming and boarding costs. I am not a tax consultant and I advise that you consult with an accountant, tax attorney, or tax advisor before taking any of the following actions that I am offering for your consideration. If you think the circumstances apply to you, you may be able to save some **BIG BUCK$** on your income taxes.

- If you use your dog as a guard dog at your place of business, all the costs of maintaining your dog should be deductible as a business expense, as would any other alarm or protection system. The same should apply if you keep your dog in or near your truck to guard your equipment while you are on the job. Avoid keeping your dog inside a vehicle when you are not present to prevent the possibility of heat stroke.

- If you deduct the costs of maintaining an office in your home, and your dog guards your home, the dog's expenses might also qualify as a deductible expense.

- If you have a seeing eye dog, all expenses would be deductible as a medical expense. Additionally, if you raise a dog for a charitable organization that trains dogs for blind people, or people with a hearing loss, your expenses may be deductible as a charitable contribution if you later donate the dog to the charitable organization.

▸ The expenses of keeping a cat, or cats, in a place of business for mouse and rat control should also be legitimate tax deductible business expenses.

Some medical problems of dogs and cats are so similar to the same medical problem in humans that it is possible to take advantage of medical products available for people. Inexpensive urine glucose test strips or test papers, available in most pharmacies, can be used if your pet has been diagnosed as having diabetes. For cats with urinary problems, litmus paper, available in pharmacies or chemical supply houses, will give you an inexpensive way to monitor your cat's urine acidity.

If your pet frequently travels by air, you will need a health certificate from your veterinarian. The best time to get this certificate is when your pet is being vaccinated by a veterinarian who includes a free examination when giving vaccinations. Airlines differ in the length of time they consider a health certificate to be valid, so be sure to call the airlines in advance to see what their rules are. If your pet travels by air infrequently, you can save money by renting an approved carrier instead of buying one and then trying to figure out where to store it after the trip is over.

CHAPTER 14:

CLIENT DISSATISFACTION

There may be a time when you are dissatisfied with your veterinarian. Feelings of dissatisfaction may be caused by many different things. Some clients may feel that they were financially cheated by their veterinarian, and others may feel that they were treated in a rude and uncaring manner. The most common causes of client dissatisfaction are when a client feels the results of the treatment were less than anticipated, or feels that the charges were higher than anticipated, causing financial shock. Most dissatisfaction can be traced back to a lack of communication between the veterinarian and the pet owner.

If the medical results are less than you anticipated, you may be dealing with a fact of medicine. Not all patients, whether they are cats, dogs, or people, respond the same way to the same disease or injury. Most veterinarians are very careful to avoid giving the impression that they are guaranteeing or promising certain results. A veterinarian, for example, can do an excellent job setting and stabilizing a broken leg, but has no control over the actual healing process which involves many cellular changes that occur within the body itself. If you feel that the results of the treatment were less than anticipated because your veterinarian made a mistake or used poor judgment, you do have recourse at several different levels, including taking legal action. Veterinarians carry malpractice insurance for a reason—like anyone else, they make mistakes.

If you feel the charges are higher than anticipated or that your veterinarian has taken an unfair advantage of you, you also have recourse. If you ask for an estimate before your veterinarian starts treatment you should never be surprised by the final bill. When your veterinarian gives you an estimate, he or she will almost never go beyond the scope of the estimate without contacting you first for permission. The only exception would be in a life threatening emergency when there is not enough time to contact you. In these cases, your veterinarian is hopefully anticipating that, if you had been contacted, you would have given your permission for the additional treatment. You, however, are not obligated to pay for those extra charges if you feel you would not have given permission for such additional treatment. While discussing your pet's case with your veterinarian, you need to carefully avoid making such statements as, "do everything possible," or, "money is no problem." In emergency situations, pet owners sometimes say these things to impress their veterinarian with the importance they place on their pet's life, but such statements can be misunderstood to mean that there is no limit on what you are willing and able to pay for veterinary services.

$ **TIP:** *If your veterinarian takes it upon himself or herself to do more than you authorized, either verbally or in writing, you are not responsible for the extra charges.*

Financial shock is a common cause for client dissatisfaction, and can occur whenever there is a lack of communication between a veterinarian and a client. Financial shock can occur when, after paying the estimated bill of $500. at an emergency clinic, you discover your pet still has a broken leg. The explanation you receive is that the surgery fee on the estimate was for suturing the skin wounds and you assumed it included fixing the broken leg. Financial shock can occur when your pet dies during a long, complicated, and expensive surgery, and you discover that you are expected to pay the entire bill, including the surgery fee. Financial shock can occur when your pet is still sick after a week in the hospital. Your veterinarian feels that the proper treatment saved your pet's life, but you feel that, for the cost, your pet should be absolutely perfect. Financial shock almost always occurs if you fail to ask for an estimate, if you get caught in a financial spiral, or if you make decisions based on emotions instead of your financial ability to pay a certain amount. Whenever financial shock occurs, client dissatisfaction is likely to occur, and there are some guidelines that you might want to follow and some actions that you might want to take, both of which you need to plan for in advance.

I recommend that you call your veterinarian's office for the final bill total before you go there to pick up your pet. If the final bill is more than a few dollars over the estimate you were given, ask for an explanation. This allows your veterinarian and staff time to review the bill and adjust the charges without anyone having to express anger or become overly defensive. If the explanation and/or fee adjustment is satisfactory to you, then you can go to your veterinarian's facility, pay the bill, and take your pet home.

If the explanation for the excess charges is not satisfactory, and if no adjustment is forthcoming, you need to get your pet out of the veterinary facility,

preferably without paying the disputed charges until you have received a proper and acceptable explanation. If you have a charge account with your veterinarian you can simply charge the entire amount and then pay everything except the disputed amount until the problem has been resolved. If you have no charge account, but are a long term client, you may be permitted to charge the unexpected portion. You can then withhold payment until you receive a satisfactory explanation. The easiest and least stressful way is to pay the entire bill with a credit card that will reverse the charges in disputed bills. When you write the credit card company they will take the amount you paid off your credit card bill until the dispute has been resolved.

If your dispute has gotten to the point where your veterinarian refuses to adjust for the charges in excess of the estimate, and refuses to allow you to take your pet home without full payment, you will need to take some type of action to resolve the dispute. In order to take further action you will need to have copies of your pet's medical records, at least the medical records concerning the disputed fees, and financial records such as estimates and itemized bills. Ask for these copies immediately upon arriving to pick up your pet from the veterinary facility. If there is no copy machine available, ask the receptionist to make a hand copy for you or make a hand copy yourself and then ask the receptionist to initial each page. There is one final consideration concerning the amount of your bill. If you feel your veterinarian overcharged you and you failed to ask for an estimate, there is probably very little action you can take as long as the fees charged were usual and customary in your geographical location. While I hate to keep repeating this advice, you need to protect yourself by always getting an estimate before you authorize treatment for your pet. If your veterinarian or veterinarian's receptionist fails to offer an estimate, ask for one before authorizing treatment.

If you are ever dissatisfied, the first level of recourse is your veterinarian. As stated earlier, most client dissatisfaction is caused by a lack of communication between the client and the veterinarian. If you were given an estimate and were then charged an amount considerably over the estimate, without being contacted for permission first, most veterinarians will adjust the bill. If your veterinarian refuses to make any adjustment or, if you were charged the estimated amount but the results were not as you anticipated, you may have to take your complaint to the next level. Remember, although a veterinarian's actions undergo little or no peer review, veterinarians are still responsible for their actions.

After discussing any complaints you have with your veterinarian and not achieving a satisfactory resolution, the next level of recourse is a veterinary medical association. Most veterinarians belong to such an association, either at the local, regional, state, or national level. Many veterinarians display their membership certificates in their facility. If you send a letter to any of these organizations, outlining in detail what has occurred and what your opinion is, you will receive a prompt response. A letter will be sent to you acknowledging receipt of your letter and telling you that action has been initiated. Simultaneously, a letter will be sent to your veterinarian listing your complaint, giving your side of the dispute, and asking your veterinarian to respond by giving the pertinent medical facts from the patient records and his or her side of the dispute. When your veterinarian responds, the facts of the case, and both points of view, will be reviewed by veterinarians skilled in these matters. After review, the association will send a letter to both you and your veterinarian, detailing the findings of the review.

If the letter you receive from the veterinary medical association is not satisfactory, or if your veterinarian does not belong to any associations having such review procedures available, the next step is to write the same letter to the Board of Veterinary Medicine in your State (see appendix B). All veterinarians, in all States, must be licensed by their State to practice veterinary medicine. The actions taken by the State Board are very similar to the actions taken by association review boards, except the State Board can take disciplinary action against the veterinarian if the facts of the case warrant such action. State Boards have the power to suspend or cancel the licenses of veterinarians.

The last level of recourse, if the above steps have not given you satisfaction, is to take appropriate legal action against the veterinarian. You can either do this in small claims court if the amount of money is below a certain level, or, after hiring a lawyer, the case can be taken to the superior court level.

When you are confident that your dissatisfaction was caused by errors made by your veterinarian, report such dissatisfaction to your local Better Business Bureau or some other consumer protection agency. They will ask your veterinarian for an explanation. If your veterinarian's explanation to the bureau or agency is satisfactory, no action will be taken, but if no satisfactory answer to your complaint is received, your complaint will be recorded, and given to others who call for information about the veterinarian or veterinary facility. No veterinarian can practice without eventually having a dissatisfied client, but most disputes can be resolved, usually to the client's financial advantage, during the client/veterinarian discussion. Typically, a veterinarian would rather make whatever adjustment is necessary and keep you as a client, than keep the dollars in dispute and have you find another doctor for your pet.

APPENDIX A

The following is a list of State Poison Control Centers. There are probably others in each State, possibly quite close to where you live. The State office can tell you where they are or you can look in your telephone book white pages.

DIRECTORY OF POISON CONTROL CENTERS

Alabama

Department of Public Health
Montgomery, AL 36117
(205) 832-3194

Alaska

Department of Health and
Social Services
Juneau, AK 99811
(907) 465-3100

Arizona

College of Pharmacy
University of Arizona
Tucson, AZ 85724
(602) 626-6016 or(800) 362-0101

Arkansas

University of Arkansas
Medical Science Campus
Little Rock, AR 72201
(501) 661-6161

California

Department of Health Services
Sacramento, CA 95814
(916) 322-4336

Colorado

Department of Health
Denver, CO 80220
(303) 320-8476

Connecticut

University of Connecticut
Health Center
Farmington, CT 06032
(203) 674-3456

Delaware

Wilmington Medical Center
Delaware Division
Wilmington, DE 19801
(302) 655-3389

District of Columbia

Department of Human Services
Washington, DC 20009
(202) 673-6741 or(202) 673-6736

Florida

Department of Health and
Emergency Medical Services
Tallahassee, FL 32301
(904) 487-1566

Georgia

Department of Human Resources
Atlanta, GA 30308
(404) 894-5170

Hawaii

Department of Health
Honolulu, HI 96801
(808) 531-7776

Idaho

Department of Health and Welfare
Boise, ID 83701
(208) 334-2241

Illinois

Div. of Emergency Medical
Services and Highway Safety
Springfield, IL 62761
(217) 785-2080

Indiana

State Board of Health
Indianapolis, IN 46206
(317) 633-0332

Iowa

Department of Health
Des Moines, IA 50319
(515) 281-4964

Kansas

Department of Health and
Environment
Topeka, KS 66620
(913) 862-9360 Ext. 451

Kentucky

Department for Human Resources
Frankfort, KY 40601
(502) 564-3970

Louisiana

Emergency Medical Services of
Louisiana
Baton Rouge, LA 70801
(504) 342-2600

Maine

Maine Poison Control Center
Portland, ME 04102
(207) 871-2950

Maryland

Maryland Poison Information
Center
University of Maryland
School of Pharmacy
Baltimore, MD 21201
(301) 528-7604

Massachusetts

Department of Public Health
Boston, MA 02111
(617) 727-2700

Michigan

Department of Public Health
Lansing, MI 48909
(517) 373-1406

Minnesota

State Department of Health
Minneapolis, MN 55404
(612) 296-5281

Mississippi

State Board of Health
Jackson, MS 39205
(601) 354-6660

Missouri

Missouri Division of Health
Jefferson City, MO 65102
(314) 751-2713

Montana

Department of Health
Montana Poison Control
Cogswell Building
Helena, MT 59620
(406) 449-3895 or (800) 525-5042

Nebraska

Department of Health
Lincoln, NE 68502
(402) 471-2122

Nevada

Department of Human Resources
Carson City, NV 86710
(702) 885-4750

New Hampshire

New Hampshire Poison Center
2 Maynard Street
Hanover, NH 03755
(603) 643-4000

New Jersey

Department of Health, Accident
Prevention and Poison Control
Trenton, NJ 08625
(609) 292-5666

New Mexico

New Mexico Poison, Drug,
and Medical Crisis Center
University of New Mexico
Albuquerque, NM 87131
(505) 843-2551 or (800) 432-6866

New York

Department of Health
Albany, NY 12237
(518) 474-3785

North Carolina

Duke University Medical Center
Durham, NC 27710
(919) 684-8111

North Dakota

Department of Health
Bismarck, ND 58505
(701) 224-2388

Ohio

Department of Health
Columbus, OH 43216
(614) 166-5100

Oklahoma

Oklahoma Poison Control
P.O. Box 26307
Oklahoma City, OK 73126
(405) 271-5454 or (800) 522-4611

Oregon

Oregon Poison Control
University of Oregon
Portland, OR 97201
(503) 225-8968 or (800) 452-7165

Pennsylvania

Division of Epidemiology
Department of Health
P.O. Box 90
Harrisburg, PA 17108
(717) 787-2307

Rhode Island

Rhode Island Poison Control
Rhode Island Hospital
593 Eddy Street
Providence, RI 02902
(401) 277-5727

South Carolina

Department of Health and
Environmental Control
Columbia, SC 29201
(803) 758-5654

South Dakota

Department of Health
Pierre, SD 57501
(605) 773-3361

Tennessee

Department of Public Health
Div. of Emergency Services
Nashville, TN 37216
(615) 741-2407

Texas

Department of Health
Div. of Occupational Health
Austin, TX 78756
(512) 458-7254

Utah

Utah Department of Health
Div. of Family Health Services
Salt Lake City, UT 84113
(801) 533-6161

Vermont

Department of Health
Burlington, VT 05401
(802) 862-5701

Virginia

Bureau of Emergency Medical
Services
Richmond, VA 23219
(804) 786-5188

Washington

Department of Social and
Health Services
Seattle, WA 98115
(206) 522-7478

West Virginia

Department of Health
Charleston, WV 25305
(304) 348-2971

Wisconsin

Department of Health
Division of Health
Madison, WI 53701
(608) -267-7174

Wyoming

Office of Emergency Medical
Services
Department of Health
Cheyenne, WY 82001
(307) 777-7955

APPENDIX B

STATE BOARDS OF VETERINARY MEDICINE

All veterinarians are licensed by their State's Veterinary Board. You may write to these Boards by addressing your correspondance to: State of _____, Veterinary Board, and using the following addresses:

Alabama

P.O. Box 1767
Decatur, AL 35602
(205) 353-3544

Alaska

P.O. Box D
Juneau, AK 99811
(907) 465-3035

Arizona

1645 West Jefferson, Rm. 410
Phoenix, AZ 85007
(602) 542-3093

Arkansas

P.O. Box 5497
Little Rock, AR 72215
(501) 224-2836

California

1420 Howe Ave., Suite 6
Sacramento, CA 95825
(916) 920-7662

Colorado

1560 Broadway, Suite 1310
Denver, CO 80202
(303) 894-7755

Connecticut

150 Washington St.
Hartford, CT 06106
(203) 566-1039

Delaware

P.O. Box 1401
Dover, DE 19903
(302) 739-4522

District of Columbia

614 H Street NW, Room 923
Washington, DC 20001
(202) 727-8030

Florida

1940 North Monroe St.
Tallahassee, FL 32399
(904) 487-1820

Georgia

166 Pryor St., SW
Atlanta, GA 30303

Hawaii

Box 3469
Honolulu, HI 96801
(808) 586-2708

Idaho

P.O. Box 7249
Boise, ID 83707
(208) 334-3962

Illinois

320 W. Washington
Springfield, IL 62786
(217) 782-8556

Indiana

402 W. Washington, Rm. 041
Indianapolis IN 46204
(317) 233-4407

Iowa

Wallace Building, 2nd Floor
Des Moines, IA 50319
(515) 281-5305

Kansas

North Star Route
Lakin, KS 67860
(316) 355-6358

Kentucky

P.O. Box 456
Frankfurt, KY 40602
(502) 564-3296

Louisiana

P.O. Box 15191
Baton Rouge, LA 70895
(504) 924-6354

Maine

State House Station #35
Augusta, ME 04333
(207) 582-8723

Maryland

50 Harry S. Truman Parkway
Annapolis, MD 21401
(310) 841-5862

Massachusetts

100 Cambridge St., Room 1516
Boston, MA 02202
(617) 727-3080

Michigan

P.O. Box 30018
Lansing, MI 48909
(517) 373-2179

Minnesota

2700 University Ave. West Rm. 102
St Paul, MN 55114
(612) 642-0597

Mississippi

209 S. Lafayette St.
Starkville, MS 39759
(601) 324-0235

Missouri

P.O. Box 633
Jefferson City, MO 65102
(314) 751-0031

Montana

Arcade Building, Lower Level
111 N. Last Chance Gulch
Helena, MT 59620
(406) 444-5436

Nebraska

P.O. Box 95007
Lincoln, NE 68509
(402) 471-2115

Nevada

1005 Terminal Way, Suite 246
Reno, NV 89502
(702) 322-9422

New Hampshire

Caller Box 2042
Concord, NH 03302
(603) 271-3706

New Jersey

P.O. Box 45020
Newark, NJ 07101
(201) 648-2841

New Mexico

1650 University Blvd. N.E.
Albuquerque, NM 87102
(505) 841-9112

New York

Room 3043
Cultural Education Center
Albany, NY 12230
(518) 474-3867

North Carolina

P.O. Box 12587
Raleigh, NC 27605
(919) 733-7686

North Dakota

600 East Blvd. J-Wing
1st Floor
Bismark, ND 58505
(701) 224-2655

Ohio

77 South High Street
16th Floor
Columbus, OH 43226
(614) 644-5281

Oklahoma

P.O. Box 18256
Oklahoma City, OK 73154
(405) 843-0843

Oregon

P.O. Box 231
Portland, OR 97207
(503) 229-5286

Pennsylvania

Box 2649
Harrisburg, PA 17105
(717) 783-1389

Rhode Island

3 Capital Hill, Rm. 104
Providence, RI 02908
(401) 277-2827

South Carolina

P.O. Box 11293
Columbia, SC 29221
(803) 253-4128

South Dakota

411 S. Fort Street
Pierre, SD 57501
(605) 773-3321

Tennessee

283 Plus Park Blvd.
Nashville, TN 37217
(615) 367-6225

Texas

1946 South IH-35 #306
Austin, TX 78704
(512) 447-1183

Utah

P.O. BOX 45802
Salt Lake City, UT 84145
(801) 530-6628

Vermont

109 State Street
Montpelier, VT 05609
(802) 828-2875

Virginia

1601 Rolling Hills Drive
Richmond, VA 23229
(804) 662-9915

Washington

1300 S.E. Quince
Olympia, WA 98504
(206) 586-6355

West Virginia

712 McCorkle Ave.
South Charleston, WV 25303
(304) 348-2016

Wisconsin

P.O. Box 8935
Madison, WI 53708
(608) 266-2811

Wyoming

Herschlier Building
Cheyenne, WY 82002
(307) 777-7515

APPENDIX C

COLLEGES AND UNIVERSITIES OF VETERINARY MEDICINE
UNITED STATES AND CANADA

The following are the universities and colleges of veterinary medicine and the main phone number of each school. When you are calling for information, or to make an appointment, ask for the small animal clinic receptionist.

Auburn University
College of Veterinary Medicine
AL, 36849
(205) 844-4546

University of California
School of Veterinary Medicine
Davis, CA 95616
(916) 752-1360

Colorado State University
College of Veterinary Medicine
Ft. Collins, CO 80523
(303) 491-7051

Cornell University
College of Veterinary Medicine
Ithaca, NY 14853
(607) 253-3000

University of Florida
College of Veterinary Medicine
Gainesville, FL 32610
(904) 392-2381

University of Georgia
College of Veterinary Medicine
Athins, GA 30602
(404) 542-3461

University of Illinois
College of Veterinary Medicine
Urbana, IL 61801
(217) 333-2760

Iowa State University
College of Veterinary Medicine
Ames, IA 50011
(515) 294-1242

Kansas State University
College of Veterinary Medicine
Manhattan, KA 66506
(913) 532-6011

Louisana State University
School of Veterinary Medicine
Baton Rouge, LA 70803
(504) 346-3200

Michigan State University
College of Veterinary Medicine
East Lansing, MI 48824
(517) 355-6509

The University of Minnesota
College of Veterinary Medicine
St. Paul, MN 55108
(612) 624-9227

Mississippi State University
College of Veterinary Medicine
Mississippi State, MS 39762
(601) 325-3432

University of Missouri
College of Veterinary Medicine
Columbia, MO 65211
(314) 882-3877

University of Montreal
Faculty of Veterinary Medicine
Saint Hyacinthe, Quebec
Canada J2S 7C6

North Carolina State University
College of Veterinary Medicine
4700 Hillsborough St.
Raleigh, NC 27606
(919) 829-4200

The Ohio State University
College of Veterinary Medicine
Columbus, OH 43210
(614) 292-1171

Oklahoma State University
College of Veterinary Medicine
Stillwater, OK 74078
(405) 744-6648

Ontario Veterinary College
University of Guelph
Guelph, Ontario
Canada N1G 2W1

Oregon State University
College of Veterinary Medicine
Corvallis, OR 97331
(503) 737-2141

University of Pennsylvania
School of Veterinary Medicine
3800 Spruce St.
Philadelphia, PA 19104
(215) 898-5438

University of Prince Edward Island
Atlantic Veterinary College
Charlottetown, Prince Edward Island
Canada C1A 4P3

Purdue University
School of Veterinary Medicine
West Lafayette, IN 47907
(317) 494-0781

University of Saskatchewan
College of Veterinary Medicine
Saskatoon, Saskatchewan
Canada S7N 0W0

University of Tennessee
College of Veterinary Medicine
Knoxville, TN 37901
(615) 974-7262

Texas A & M University
College of Veterinary Medicine
College Station, TX 77843
(409) 845-5051

Tufts University
School of Veterinary Medicine
200 Westboro Rd.
North Grafton, MA 01536
(508) 839-5302

Tuskegee University
School of Veterinary Medicine
Tuskegee, AL 36088
(205) 727-8011

Virginia-Maryland Regional
College of Veterinary Medicine
Blacksburg, VA 24061
(703) 231-7666

Washington State University
College of Veterinary Medicine
Pullman, WA 99164
(509) 335-9515

University of Wisconsin-Madison
School of Veterinary Medicine
Madison, WI 53706
(608) 263-6716